BOTH/AND

ESSAYS BY TRANS AND
GENDER-NONCONFORMING
WRITERS OF COLOR

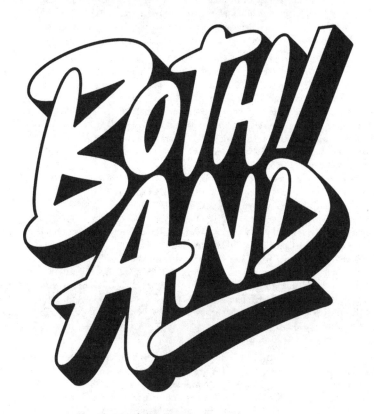

EDITED BY **DENNE MICHELE NORRIS**
WITH **ELECTRIC LITERATURE**

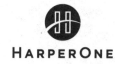

HarperOne

An Imprint of HarperCollins*Publishers*

HarperCollins books may be purchased for educational, business, or sales promotional use. For information, please email the Special Markets Department at SPsales@harpercollins.com.

harpercollins.com

FIRST EDITION

Designed by Yvonne Chan

Library of Congress Cataloging-in-Publication Data has been applied for.

ISBN 978-0-06-341437-2

25 26 27 28 29 LBC 5 4 3 2 1

For the gworls, the bois, and everyone in between and beyond.

"I'm still fucking here!"

—Miss Major Griffin-Gracy

CONTENTS

COMING TO LIGHT

INTRODUCTION

DENNE MICHELE NORRIS

In the early aughts—when I was in high school—my friends and I often chose Claire's as our meetup location at the mall. We perused the accessories and sometimes could even afford to buy a trendy charm bracelet or puka shell necklace. One humid summer night in Cleveland, a copper armband caught my eye. It was the kind of thing I imagined Cleopatra might have worn, curled several times around the upper arm, each end adorned with the ruby-eyed head of a snake. The ornament looked out of place hanging from a shelf in Claire's, as out of place as I felt standing there in a polo shirt and loose cargo shorts, gawking at it. My friends were running late, so I tried it on, walking around the store, glancing in every mirror. After a few minutes I stood in front of where I'd found it, considering if I'd really wear it if I purchased it.

"It's fine for you to try that on as long as you don't buy it." A saleswoman had crept up behind me. She was Black, with graying hair pulled back into a tight bun, and she wore stockings, and the sensible, kitten-heeled shoes of a woman who never missed her Sunday church service. I didn't know her, and yet I knew her very well.

"I'm sorry?"

"You wouldn't actually buy that. You're not a girl; it's not for you."

She had clocked me.

"No, ma'am, I guess I'm not."

I placed the armband into her outstretched hand and rushed from the store, my eyes lowered to the ground as I frantically texted my friends to meet me elsewhere. I was angry and embarrassed, but mostly I felt exposed. I'd been standing by myself in a store meant for teenage girls in a suburban mall in middle America. I typically felt invisible, but with one glance, one comment, this woman let me know that she could see me for what I was—and what I wasn't.

A year later, a friend and I visited a different mall, a fancier mall, one that didn't even have a Claire's. We walked around, he and I, deep in conversation about sexual identity and stereotypes, when he asked me, quite calmly, if I had ever considered the idea that I might actually be a girl—one who'd simply been born into the wrong body.

I considered his question. His tone was gentle, but his query was sharp, pointed, and it lodged itself inside of me. I was aware of trans people's existence—because of the *T* in the acronym *LGBT*, and because I'd seen episodes of *The Nanny* and *Will and Grace*— but they had always been, to me, more theoretical than real.

Being "trans" seemed an unthinkable way to move through the world. I was already Black, and gay, and the son of a well-known Baptist minister. I was a high school senior who had somehow managed to survive at a deeply conservative all-boys prep school. Soon I would be a freshman at a progressive liberal arts college outside Philadelphia. I had worked hard in school, convinced that leaving Cleveland and never looking back was the only answer if I wanted to live my best Black queer life. This college—a campus where *The Princeton Review* said it was easier to come out as queer than as a Republican—was my reward. I wanted to step into the freedom of the real world and distance myself from the context in which I was raised. I was not looking for further marginalization.

I told my friend that I was not transgender, but his question punctured me like a bullet that wouldn't, or couldn't, be removed.

//

I first had the idea for an essay series centering trans and gender-nonconforming writers of color in fall 2021. I had recently been named the editor in chief of *Electric Literature*, a groundbreaking digital literary magazine with an annual readership of more than three million. A few months earlier, I'd publicly disclosed my identity as a trans woman, something I'd been preparing to do for two years in response to a question I'd been asking myself for sixteen years. When I was named to this new role, I was widely celebrated as the first Black, openly transgender woman to helm a major literary publication.

Around this time, the comedian Dave Chappelle released a new Netflix special, *The Closer*, in which he pitted the Black community and the LGBTQ community against each other, arguing that queer white people are better off in contemporary American society than Black people and often participate in the racist marginalization of Black people. The role played by different marginalized groups in each other's oppression deserves a richly considered and nuanced conversation, but instead, Chappelle completely erased the existence of those who live at the intersection of Black and queer identities.

Around this same time, Chimamanda Ngozi Adichie published an essay that doubled down on an evasive response she gave when asked whether or not a trans woman is a woman: "My feeling is that trans women are trans women." This puzzled me. As a woman who claims to be in alliance with the LGBTQ+ community, her choice to write the essay felt like an intentional antitrans dog whistle to her global army of supporters, many of whom are self-identified TERFs (trans-exclusionary radical feminists).

But Chappelle infuriated me. The popularity of his special, and the conversation it ignited, remained a major talking point in news media for weeks. Netflix defended the special, resulting in a walkout by the company's trans employees. Over weeks of social media and news media discourse, what I noticed was this: For all the dialogue surrounding trans identity, the loudest voices in this conversation were never trans people and, in particular, were never trans people of color. We were the existential center of a cultural boiling point—and our voices were almost nowhere to be found.

From my fury was born *Both/And*, a series of fifteen essays published online by *Electric Literature*, with the goal of elevating emerging trans and gender-nonconforming writers of color to a national literary platform. But there was one key distinction—these writers would have the unique opportunity to be edited by a trans writer of color. *Electric Literature* quickly fundraised to support the series, meeting and then exceeding our goal in just one week, proving that writers and readers alike were hungry for these essays. The popularity of the series, which was published on electricliterature.com in 2023, as well as the ever-growing far-right political targeting of the LGBTQ+ community, further proves how necessary these essays are.

Last year Donald Trump won the 2024 presidential election, during which Republicans spent hundreds of millions of dollars on antitrans ads. As I watched the results, my heart fell from my chest. I knew what was coming, and predictably, less than twelve hours later, I tuned in to morning shows where I saw political pundits—from both parties—blaming the trans community for the election results. Early analysis saw folks saying that the Democratic Party was out of touch with the majority of American voters, that the party was too woke, that American families didn't want grown men playing sports against little girls. The absurdity of that statement aside, I kept thinking to myself, *But I'm an American voter, too.*

What followed was a profound sense of displacement, politically speaking. While my values are progressive, I have always been a voter motivated by pragmatism and harm reduction. I was raised in a Black, middle-class family of churchgoers by parents born between the Silent Generation and the Baby Boomers. I was raised to vote in every election. And I was raised to vote without attaching a grave sense of preciousness to that vote. It wasn't necessary to agree with everything my chosen political candidate said, in part because voting wasn't supposed to be the sum of my political engagement. It was a chess move, a means to an end, and it was the bare minimum. More simply put, I have always been a registered voter, and I have always voted for the Democratic ticket. Given my values, this means I have also, always, held a deep sense of frustration at the party's continued pursuit of moderate white voters.

Being Black, and being queer, I have always worried that when it comes to policy, measures that affirmed and protected my existence would end up on the chopping block. And very often, that's exactly what happened. But in recent years, public opinion has shifted. Marriage equality, for instance, has been legal for nearly a decade, and folks have largely realized that their heterosexual marriages were never in danger. Perhaps it was the optimism of youth or the stability of democracy, but I never looked into the future fearing what it held for me or my community. Yet when faced with the possibility of a rebooted Trump administration, I felt strongly that Kamala Harris needed to win if I was to maintain any sense of safety.

Whenever progress is made, there's corresponding backlash. Right now we live in a time of escalated targeting of the LGBTQ+ community, and yet we stand on the precipice of an even darker era. Being a writer, I turn to literature in times of darkness—the writing of it and, more important, the reading of it. In the face of a political class that, at best, hesitates to stand beside us and, at worst, works to bring about our ruin, I introduce you to the brilliant writers in this anthology, all of whom live at the fraught intersection of race and gender identity.

Each of these essays is a wonder, something taken from the heart of its writer and flung, with delicious abandon, into this world. Each essay leaves an echo, promising to reverberate inside the reader. There is Akwaeke Emezi, who meditates on what it means to be beautiful across gender, and Tanaïs, who writes about the fantasy of making feverish love to another femme to mark the occasion of a landmark birthday. Meredith Talusan remembers a casual hookup that awakened the woman within, and Gabrielle Bellot travels to Hawaii with her wife, where the eruption of a volcano inspires her inner goddess. These are just a handful of the essays that turn their gaze inward and backward, straddling—and sometimes weaving together—what it means to be man or woman, masc or femme.

There are also essays that turn their gaze fearlessly forward, conjuring the sort of tender, loving future we so rarely get to live. Zeyn Joukhadar considers what it means to be part of a future their ancestors never lived to see. Kaia Ball dreams about their estranged father coming out as trans and finding a way to accept them. Jonah Wu brings the reader along as he jumps off the proverbial cliff into the world of hormone replacement therapy, embracing a more masculine future. And A. L. Major considers the cost of creating the life, and family, of their choosing.

Historically, trans people have been forced to imagine, or conjure, representation of ourselves into existing narratives that never sought to include us, often using the stories and fictional lives of canonically cishet characters as foundations for possible trans stories. *Both/And* is unabashed in its portrayal of the fullness of our lives. These essays consider imagination and fantasy as real-world liberation, the heightened visibility and invisibility of trans bodies, trans joy, laughter and love, and trans rage, revenge, and loss.

At *Electric Literature*, we believe that literature has the power to shape public consciousness. Storytelling breaks down barriers in numerous ways, perhaps the most powerful being the building of empathy. My community is under vicious attack on every level, but we refuse to disappear, and I refuse to allow our stories and our lives to be erased. The time is now for trans and gender-nonconforming writers of color to amplify our own voices on our own terms. While the culture is obsessed with us, that obsession has been weaponized in an effort to legislate us out of existence. But it simply won't work, because we're already here. We've *been* here, telling our stories in our own words, our voices rising to the rafters, ringing so loud that we're impossible to ignore.

SELFHOOD

OBJECT LESSONS

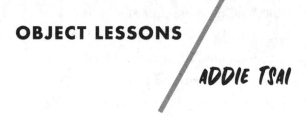

ADDIE TSAI

As a twin you know too well what it means
to have your embodiment bound to another,
whether to run from sameness or to cling to it.

From as far back as you can remember until you left home at eighteen, your Ba has starred in Mandarin stage dramas he produced
with his Taiwanese friends as part of a nonprofit theater company,
the first to produce a Mandarin-language play in the American
South. Because of this company, you've watched your Ba DJ for
Chinese dance parties, direct a Vietnamese Elvis impersonator
to offer you a plastic rose as you stood next to the stage, command the floor with your stepmother in a rousing paso doble. As
teenagers, you and your twin are occasionally asked to join in—to
open a night of folk dance as ghostly doubles inching across the
stage behind a scrim; to sing the karaoke hit 九百九十九朵玫瑰
at the Chinese Community Center's yearly white elephant party;
to squeeze into *qipaos* and strut the catwalk for a fashion show;

to stand or charge while holding makeshift spears as soldiers in a Mandarin adaptation of *King Lear*—accompanied by eyeliner mustaches and foam armor painted silver and gridded black.

When your brother and twin are not directly asked to participate, they couldn't be less interested in the endless hours of rehearsals, the plays in a language you're never encouraged to speak or understand, or even the books your Ba tells you to bring to make it through the long days and nights.

For you, this is not the case.

Your eyes burn with want, a desire released from the fear of embodiment—being called upon by the aunties to answer in stilted, unaccented Mandarin or resort to overly perfected English (the execution more exposing of your alien American ways than considered impressive for its articulation); the dreaded summoning of you and your twin to the microphone to sing Mandarin karaoke, whose words you sound out from the pinyin your father speaks while you record them in a three-ring binder; or that one time your Ba directed you to mount the stage with your violin to test the sound after your private lesson only to admonish your sadly mediocre playing on the car ride home. But watching is deliciously free, as long as you're discreet about it. Chinese eyes are usually so loud, but you have always known how to inhale all the details without being detected.

You are young, but probably older than you imagine. You sit next to your Ba as he cakes his face in greasepaint. Some roles call for shoe polish just above the cheekbones and below his uniquely deep-set eyes, a result of the Mongolian ancestry you share. His eyes have already been roughly outlined in thick black pencil. His hair is tied in a bun at the top of his head, wrapped with a square of brown fabric, to match the *changshan* he wears. While he sits in front of a small cosmetic mirror in a dressing room, he bellows in a tongue you know as intimately as your skin but that is shrouded in mystery—not unlike your Ba himself. The voice of an auntie, one of the many who remain nameless to you, ricochets back, and soon a boy your age who plays your Ba's son delivers a tube of red lipstick. It is your favorite part, watching your Ba's lips come to life like fireworks.

//

The first time you're scolded as a child for a physical act *unbecoming* of a girl is at The Clubhouse, the Montessori after-school and weekend day care where you learn to play basketball, draw, write, sew, compete in tiered-level tournaments in *Montezuma's Revenge* on Atari, and swim at the rec center pool. It's not that you want to be a boy, but it's already becoming clear to you that girls are shaped in ways that aggravate the dissonance between you, a distance already carved by your not-quite-whiteness, your fractured divorced home, your wild and brazen white mother, your Taiwanese NASA-engineer-by-day-actor-by-night father. You're not quite like the boys, either, but they don't mind your company as long as you're not precious or overly sensitive. Your Ba never handles you with kid gloves, that's for sure. You *are* tenderhearted, as your Ba loves reminding you when his harsh tongue immediately brings you to tears, but that softness is saved only for him.

On one Saturday morning at The Clubhouse, you sit on the carpet with three boys so ultimately insignificant you can't even summon a guess at their names, their looks so generic white 1980s you couldn't pick them out of a group photograph. The four of you while away the time comparing moles. One rolls up the sleeve of his T-shirt. Another raises the bottom of his shorts to reveal a fuzzy dark oval on his thigh. You pull down your shorts and underwear, just an inch, to expose the brown dot, just a hair larger than a freckle, barely below your belly. It is just you and the boys, and the interaction between the three of you is innocent, sexless. Suddenly, from high above you, the shrill voice of a teacher, whose name and face have also blurred in your memory beyond recognition: *Addie!* she screams. As you hurriedly raise your waistband back up to your belly, the boys nudging you in the elbow and chuckling, shame (a word you don't yet hold) bleeds through. Perhaps this is why those boys lose their importance, their faces and names fading from view. The teacher, you grow to understand, is a thief—of your genderless innocence, your body years from ripening. You'll never feel safe with those boys again. You will lose yourself in drawing comics and writing little stories for *The Clubhouse Rally*, the stapled magazine made of xeroxed pages and cutouts and glue stick. That teacher will say nothing when one of the young men who supervises you and the other children holds you by your ankles upside down under the basketball hoop and calls you by your middle name, which you despise, over and over again, while another tickles you as you squirm and shout for them to stop. This, too, is about gender. This, too, is a thievery, but it is also a lesson you learn you are privileged to be taught only once or twice.

//

In your twenties, you ride shotgun as your best friend drives to a juke joint. He is a Black gay man from the South. You love the Sam Cooke song crooning through the speakers. When Sam whistles, so do you. Your bestie practically falls out of his seat. He tells you his mama always told his sister it wasn't polite for girls to whistle. You laugh at the idea of whistling a song being ascribed such a value as politeness. You cringe at the idea that only boys and men would be allowed such a joyous pastime. You stop. He assures you that you can continue to enjoy the song, but the moment has passed. You won't remember all of the lessons like your first one, that of the whistling, but adulthood will shower you with so many accidental thefts from so many sources that *teach* you what it means to be she. They will feel like being nicked by a knife, or a pellet from a BB gun.

Each time you are taught a lesson about the *rules* of gender, you will think back to your Ba's red mouth, his small bun. You will see his thick floral apron stretched tightly over his round belly as he fills mini pie crusts with cheesecake for your orchestra bake sales. You will revisit the time he taught your sister to dance, helped you perfect your runway walk for the qipao fashion show. A montage of all your father's roles flutter behind the eyes. Through them you have always known that the gendered body, an ever-evolving performance, is never static. You have known this outside of theory, or even language—that it is through the play of gendered embodiment that true euphoria lives.

Not once will you recall him telling you the rules and restrictions of girlhood. Not once will you recall witnessing him tell your brother how one must behave (or abstain from behaving) to be a man.

In your forties, he will tell you over *xiaolongbao* about one of his earliest roles onstage in Taiwan, as a waitress, after you ask him when acting became a serious vocation for him. No one, including your stepmother, will bat an eye at this anecdote. You understand that this is a luxury.

//

It will take some time for you to learn that this lack makes you one of the lucky ones. In many other ways, you were not dealt the easiest hand as far as childhood is concerned. But you will learn, just as you do with your own expansive, ever-shifting relationship to gender, to take the totality of your childhood by the yard like a shimmering fabric, wrap it across your face as you angle your chin up toward the sky. Only then will you find the perforations in between, what your Ba even among all his imperfections makes possible.

//

It's your first girlfriend, your only queer Asian love, who teaches you at twenty-eight how tightly wound a butch-femme dynamic can be. You're too green a queer to understand that to be her femme means that each step you take away from the hug of a fabric to your hips and breasts is inextricably tied to how masculine she can feel. As a twin you know too well what it means to have your embodiment bound to another, whether to run from sameness or to cling to it. She cringes when you throw on a pair of cargo shorts to walk the dog. You are *allowed* to embrace the essence of a tomboy, but only if it comes with lip gloss and form-fitting jeans. You're expected to turn an unknowing eye to her constant garnering of flirtation and attention from white women she doesn't find attractive, or lean in to the role of the jealous hysteric, so she can relish in embodying the macho fuckboi with swag. So long as the heat brings out the stone butch in her, the ever-available concubine in you. You'd hoped to find a haven in a fellow Asian, but instead are faced with yet another performance. Except this stage isn't the scene of queering play, the kind you'd delighted in when watching your Ba as a little babe; it's a set of rules housing a heteronormative cosplay you've never been taught.

//

Not all is lost. Although your Ba doesn't immediately make peace with your queer love held up to the light of day, he quickly comes around, unearthing from deep in his own closet queer and trans films from Asia you never knew existed. What would have changed for you if you'd found his hiding place earlier? You and your queer Asian love gleefully speculate about your Ba as you make your way through his catalog dominated by films featuring Asian trans women, often connected to theatrical performance.

You tell her about the time your Ba was cast in an independent short film as the father of a woman whose white boyfriend (who is also his co-worker) attempts to ask for her hand in marriage over a game of mah-jongg, while the father's son gathers the courage to come out. Your Ba writes the director a letter respectfully suggesting a scene for the son, in which the son applies a full face of makeup in the bathroom, letting it speak his queerness into being that his father can't silence with words. In the letter, your Ba suggests Boy George's "The Crying Game" play in the background as the son encounters his new face in the mirror, rehearsing his impending confrontation with unabashed sass.

You tell her about your Ba's admiration of *Brokeback Mountain* when it was first released, an expression so sincere he was almost brought to silence—"I was just so impressed a man from my background could make a movie like that," shaking his head in awe. You tell her that this moment, on the heels of your coming out, just a couple of years before meeting her, meant more than he could possibly know.

Your Ba's catalog, his empathic reflection, certainly beg the question, one that remains a mystery. Or perhaps, you ponder, it is even a rarer and more precious act, that a cishet Asian father can embody multiplicities. Could you imagine it?

> To accept the way in which one is lost is to be also
> found and not found in a particularly queer fashion.
> JOSÉ MUÑOZ

//

When you watch *Farewell My Concubine* with your Ba in the theater at thirteen, you don't think anything of Douzi's face softened by a pink cloud around the eyes, lips red as your Ba's from childhood, his voice the air circling the inside of a bell. His unrequited obsession with Shitou is unremarkable enough that you don't recall it in great detail. Notes of tragedy, opera, violence, love, and heartbreak ring out most clearly in your memory. A boy performing as a woman, that you remember. But just as it is in the film, you hold no awareness of what you remember as anything to reject, whether in yourself or others. And for that matter, you've met enough of your mother's gay friends to not find it a surprise that a man could love another man. But then you're fifteen, walking down the street with your white best friend, who is the daughter of a Methodist reverend. You're telling a funny story about one of your mother's closest friends, a Jewish hairdresser who runs a salon with his Latine partner. "You know," she says, interrupting your delight, "I don't agree with it." "With what?" you ask, confused. *How could you not love this story?* you think to yourself, your innocence, again, stinging with a clarity you'd prefer remained blurred in the background.

//

As far back as the Yuan dynasty, men and women cross-dressed on Chinese stages. The earliest recorded practice of *kunsheng*—women performing in male roles, also known as female men—was during the Tang dynasty. These women portrayed military male figures, demonstrating mastery of martial arts and acrobatics. During the Yuan dynasty, actresses impersonated men in intersex theater troupes, proving their ability to take on any role.

The kunsheng demonstrated that assigned gender at birth was not the primary consideration when casting roles. Theater during the Yuan period considered gender an aspect of a character illustrated through costume, gesture, historical context, and other cultural factors. Gender was then an externalization manipulated by performers—and celebrated as an aspect of performance.

When Manchurian rules banned public performances by women in the late eighteenth century, male actors cross-dressed out of necessity. Imperial Chinese society considered it improper for men and women to appear onstage together. The following century, Qing law prohibited government officials from patronizing brothels or visiting sex workers, as theater and prostitution came to be viewed as performing arts, unsuitable for women. This shift led to the creation of brothels known as *xianggong tangzi* (the house of female boys), found on most corners of Beijing in the mid-nineteenth century, where men paid to have sex with young boys impersonating female characters from Chinese opera, which flourished during the Qing dynasty (1644–1911). The boys were trained in female acting techniques, leading them ultimately to find their home in the professional theater.

Women returned to the stage in the twentieth century, but this long history of male and female impersonation never truly left Chinese opera.

MARTINI FISHER (AS PARAPHRASED)

//

Roles like the *nandan* [men who perform traditionally female theatrical roles] and the *nüxiaosheng* [young male roles performed by women] are complex and challenging because they demand the actor break through the barriers of biology and gender, and reach toward an unattainable masculine or feminine ideal.

CHEN TIAN

//

Although Taiwanese opera began in the nineteenth century, it only really developed in the twentieth century, a theatrical style that relies on women performing as men, xiaosheng, so frequently it is almost required.

EMILY FENG

//

*[Xiaosheng] represents the idealized male
image, based on a woman's viewpoint.*

JASMINE CHEN

//

*In Taiwanese opera, men perform often as
women.* Men like to be in costume, actor Chang
Min-jyun says, and be beautiful, too.

EMILY FENG

//

As a child, you wear boys' clothes out of necessity and practicality,
your Ba often dressing you in what your older brother has outworn.
When you and your twin hit teenhood, your Ba now married to a
woman, he's more conscious of occasions expecting femme attire—
like the violet frock with the velvet empire bust and satin skirt
worn to perform karaoke or the black pin-striped vest and pencil
skirt to attend an uncle's birthday party. Your hair, cut to the neck
until adolescence, is also a matter of convenience and ease, one less
task for your Ba to handle as a single parent of three children. But
in all of these cases, the clothing is stripped of essentialist attitudes
or joined behavior about what it means to be she or he. *Boys' clothes*
are simple, durable, cheaper to clean. *Girls' clothes* are attached to
pageantry but more to an attitude of the outside world. In other
words, you wear dresses to perform, or to please the aunties.

//

It will take many years for the weight of your father's lessons to seep fully into your skin. No matter how intently he tries to keep you from the outside world, it hits back hard in all its confusing violence. You spend those years volleying back and forth between the lessons of those you love, messages that carry through the generations. Sometimes you are taught these lessons by accident. A friend simply wants to vent about the weight of all their burdens. But on occasion you feel the twinge of an edge in the teaching: They resent you, you think, for having a Ba who dressed you like a boy, or a Ma who sat open-legged and talked as crassly as Roseanne Barr. And so they splatter you with all these conditions that apparently accompany this body part or that spoken octave. *How dare you,* they seem to say, *think you can be freed of this grime that has always lived on our skin?*

And so, you try to play along. You try on soft femme, high dandy. There are aspects of each you relish in—the flourish of waves and frills, colors and cosmetics; the refined line of a tailored suit and a crisp white shirt, the sharp command of a classic oxford's wooden heel. But there is always something missing in the reception of the gaze. It is almost always accompanied by all the miseducation of *she this, he that.*

It takes you some time, but one day, you finally return to that moment of your Ba, the mirror, and the lipstick.

Just like your Ba, one day, you, too, will prepare for the stage.

In early August 2022, in a swanky downtown Manhattan Airbnb, you stand in the living room before a full-length mirror hung horizontally against the wall. You wear a flirty skirt made of polyester mesh in kelly green, sprinkled with various colored beads, designed by Chloe Dao, the second winner of *Project Run-*

way, a Vietnamese American designer born and raised in Houston, where you lived most of your life and, of course, where your Ba performed all those years ago. You pair Chloe with your royal blue women's blazer from Zara, the inside lining painted with a replica of your book cover by Zach Paugh, a mixed-race Filipinx Polish Hawaiian costume designer and artist you interviewed for your queer fashion magazine. Your shoes are a holiday exclusive collaboration between JW Anderson and Converse, brightening the classic All Star sneaker into a sparkly color-block lace-up in red, green, and blue. Your calves are graced by thin knee-high nylon stockings the same shade of blue as the blazer. Across your chest is a men's short-sleeved blue floral button-down, one of your Target staples that stands the test of time and versatility. You stand before the mirror solely as a source of security and comfort, because you don't need it: You drape the multicolored floral bow tie around your collar, pull one side just an inch lower than the other, and tie it around your neck without needing to look in the reflection. You complete the look with your own red lipstick, bright green shadow, black eyeliner, and pale blush.

Onstage, you read to an audience for the first time from your second novel, *Unwieldy Creatures*. The book is a queer Asian retelling of *Frankenstein*, and its journey includes *Victor Frankenstein*, a dance theater adaptation you cocreated with a contemporary ballet choreographer a decade before, in which all that watching of your Ba's performances that you did came to life in the set, lighting, sound design, costumes, staging, movement.

Weeks before you step on your own makeshift stage before a microphone at the back patio of a bar in Brooklyn, you leave home for the first time. Your Ba asks to meet you at a restaurant in Chinatown. You share a simple, quiet meal together, mostly in comforting silence. In the parking lot afterward, he asks you to wait while he grabs something from his car. In his hands he holds a modest black bag with a thick strap. He tells you it's a unisex bag, designed for men but one women also wear. You hold back tears as you accept it from him, considering all the object lessons between this one and the one that began them all.

Holding the bag to your chest, you hope you always remember his greatest gift to you: To treat each day as an opportunity for exploration and possibility with your body, your costume, your face. To delight in the role you have chosen to play. Gender, like the stage, never expires of possibilities. You need only take your cue.

BODY TYPE 1

VANE$$A ANGÉLICA VILLARREAL

Fantasy is where I have the power to topple
tyrants and change a burning world.

On an unseasonably hot Halloween of this brutal year, that
liminal day when the veil between the living and the dead is
thinnest—and five days before Donald Trump was once again
elected president on a platform of white grievance and hate—
BioWare's long-awaited game *Dragon Age: The Veilguard* released
to a rabid fandom. Some fans like me were beyond excited, having
waited years for this next chapter of the story after *Dragon Age:
Inquisition* left us in an agonizing cliff-hanger in the *Trespasser*
downloadable content.

But the most toxic corners of the internet had already been
seething for months, enraged at the "woke" inclusion of trans
and nonbinary options and characters in the forthcoming
Dragon Age game. Despite BioWare's long history of LGBTQ
representation, popular Twitch streamers launched a vitriolic

smear campaign, posting fake documents and misleading game footage claiming that *The Veilguard* "forced" players to be transgender through an optional dialogue wheel—a claim that, upon release of the game, proved to be ragebait. (Just click the Back button.) These streamers criticized the character creator, which, as in many new games, had moved away from making players choose to play as "male" or "female" and toward a more inclusive range of "body types," allowing players to fully customize their racial and gender expressions, from hair textures to melanin content, genitals and voice, even top surgery scars—little details that, while not all visible in gameplay, exist to affirm the identity of the player. And they took issue at the inclusion of Taash, the first nonbinary companion in the history of gaming, whose story of transition is made all the more poignant as that of a Qunari warrior, belonging to a race and culture that is an allegory for Islam. These inclusions were contested on many grounds, but most strenuously as inconsistent with *Dragon Age* "lore" and the "accurate portrayal" of an imagined, or fictional, medieval history.

In fandoms, lore—specifically the adherence to "lore accuracy" and "historical accuracy"—is weaponized as a means of gatekeeping and discrediting the diversification of fantasy. The implication is that such measures amount to "forced DEI." Would-be Nicene Councils of "real" fans and self-deputized loremasters form, working to uphold the original, authentic writings of the original text as the final word and to police any interpretations that deviate from "canon." Much like evangelical Christians, with their insistence on the Bible as the final word, the lore police operate from authority, with the author viewed as something of a god. The arguments they make—*Nonbinary identity isn't possible given the strict gender roles of the Qunari culture. Trans identity politics are ahistorical. Top surgery was not possible in medieval times. Why are there top surgery scars in a world where healing potions and spells exist?*—all focus on claimed lore violations. These are used as grounds to protest the inclusion of trans and nonbinary narratives in the game.

But the existence of queer, trans, and gender-fluid people is well attested in antique and medieval history. Trans characters such as Maevaris and Krem from past *Dragon Age* games are canon, and many characters have prominent scars and prosthetics. In the case of Taash, their nonbinary identity is made all the richer *because* they are an immigrant's kid, whose dual culture allows them to define themselves outside of the strict gender roles of the Qun. In any event, *Dragon Age* is not history but *fantasy*, a genre set in an imagined world, where the stories of our present are worked out in allegory. Rather than romanticize the past, *Dragon Age* complicates fantasy, and its ambition is to stage the violent histories fantasy is rooted in: colonialism, racial oppression, enslavement, dispossession, forced conversion, rebellion. Still, the damage was done. *Dragon Age* was review-bombed on Metacritic and Steam within hours of its release and, for unknown reasons, was shut out of every category but one at the 2024 Game Awards.

The antiwoke backlash to *The Veilguard* is a microcosm of the broader culture war being fought on the national stage. Donald Trump ran his second reelection campaign on a platform of hate and disinformation, claiming that kids were being "forced" to transition their gender at school, a claim Twitch streamer Asmongold repeated on his first playthrough of *The Veilguard* when presented with optional gender-based dialogue: "There's no option not to be transgender . . . Guys, I don't know what to do! . . . Forced transgender?—this is what Donald Trump was talking about!" This controversy may seem like a tiny drop in a much bigger wave of reactionary politics, but arguably, gaming is its *origin* point, starting with Gamergate, a 2014 defamation campaign against women in the video game industry and the blueprint for sustained online harassment from internet trolls who formed the alt-right pipelines, targeted incel rage, and normalized the red pill internet. And crucially, these toxic fandoms are particularly possessive of fantasy, a genre set in a medieval European imaginary—a history before colonialism, rendered in whiteness.

Still, I was surprised at the vitriolic intensity of the backlash, especially so far ahead of release. The meteoric success of *Baldur's Gate 3* just a year earlier had seemed to mark a cultural turning point, as the game earned overwhelmingly positive reviews from even the most stalwart bigots despite its unapologetic queer and trans inclusion. I'd found a thriving commons in *Baldur's Gate* and *Dragon Age* fandoms, made up mostly of queer, trans, BIPOC, and women gamers. *The Veilguard* hadn't done anything new; other games like *Cyberpunk 2077* also allowed trans and nonbinary customization. What was the problem?

//

Just a few weeks ago, I learned of a collaborative project called the Woke Content Detector, a massive Google spreadsheet published in March 2024 and continually updated since, logging video games containing instances of so-called woke content and ranking them. A quick skim of the reasons given in the "not recommended" column range from "pro-LGBTQ+ messaging" to "pro-DEI messaging and forced diversity" and "interracial relationships." (No word on interracial relationships involving fantasy races such as elves, though—or on interspecies relationships, for that matter.) The list reads like a hysterical catalog of content triggers and grievances, sounding the alarm for other straight white men (even instances of rainbows and rainbow flags are listed), color-coded on a scale from blue (no woke content detected; recommended) to yellow (subtle messaging; informational) to red (not recommended). Needless to say, the red entries far outnumber the blue and yellow, including more than half of all the games. As of this writing, out of 1,549 games logged, this is the rating breakdown:

Not Recommended: 822 Games (53 Percent)

The "not recommended" category is the largest by far, with more than double the number of games as the other categories, including such massively popular titles as *Baldur's Gate 3*, *Elden Ring*, and even *Call of Duty: Modern Warfare*. The objections to these games mostly involve "overtly pro-LGBTQ+" themes, "DEI messaging," and "forced diversity inaccurate for the time period," but also weirdly specific complaints like "vitiligo sliders," "humanizing asylum seekers," and "shaming the patriarchy." Disabilities also do not escape notice, from representations of anxiety and wheelchair use to the promotion of COVID-19 masking and social distancing in *Tony Hawk's Pro Skater 1+2*.

Interracial relationships also trigger a "not recommended" rating. In the entry for *Until Dawn*, a complaint about a "Black male–Asian female couple" is backed up by a link to Pew Research data showing that "Asian-Black intermarriages make up less than 2% of all intermarriages," which should ostensibly stand as evidence that a relationship between a Black man and an Asian woman is unlikely. (This complaint does not appear in the review of *PGA Tour*, however, which includes a playable Tiger Woods, the son of a Black man and Asian woman.)

By far the sorest complaint, however, is the inclusion of queer and trans characters, identities, options, and themes, especially in character creation menus. In recent years, role-playing games have moved away from involving the choice to play as either a "male" or "female" character and shifted toward offering a range of body types—some more feminine-presenting, others more masculine-presenting, with gender identity, voice, pronouns, and genitalia as separate options altogether. The way women's representation has also become much more inclusive has incensed antiwoke gamers. A search for keywords across the list reveals a whopping 995 instances of *LGBTQ*, 77 instances of *trans*, 106 instances of *gender*, 210 instances of *pronouns*, and 237 instances of *nonbinary*. In the character creation menus of newer role-playing games, the shift toward a more trans-inclusive choice of "body type," with separate options for gender identity and genitals, has drawn the most ire.

Informational: 321 Games (21 Percent)

Although most of the games here are coded yellow rather than red, this category is simply a continuation to a lesser degree of the "not recommended" category, listing games such as *Red Dead Redemption 2*, *Fallout*, and *The Witcher 3: Wild Hunt*. It's also arguably the most fascinating section, logging "minor" instances of wokeness and homoerotic "subtleties" that do more to reveal the hidden politics of the *authors* and their fragility when they see anything that does not conform to the gated community they've made of gaming. The flags in this section range from effeminate male characters to feminist non-playable characters and from mixed-race families to genderless cats that can be romanced, married, and bred regardless of gender—not to mention the magical gender-swap coffin in *Dark Souls II.* (Even the *Police Quest Collection* from 1987 is flagged for containing a "minor gay NPC" and a "cross-dresser.") The compilers of the list even "out" closeted games—a mere hint of homoeroticism, or an offhand comment made by a developer, prompts the woke content detectives to find damning evidence of hidden gayness. For example, in the entry for *BioShock,* the review reads:

> Contains LGBTQ+ messaging. According to creative director Ken Levine, the minor NPC Sander Cohen is gay. In-game audio logs allude to possible homosexual interactions. Pro- or anti- is unclear.

The mere *intent* to include homosexuality, found in unused dialogue recordings mined from audio logs, is enough to warrant a content flag.

Recommended: 403 Games (26 Percent)

So what's good? What games *do* the Woke Content Detectors recommend? A strange collection, endorsing such hard-hitting titles as *Putt-Putt Joins the Parade* (1992) and *Chicken Invaders 1–5*—but also, perhaps most tellingly, the falsification of data, earning the first games in popular franchises, such as *The Witcher* (queer sex; monster sex), *Final Fantasy* (gender fluidity, light communism), and *BioShock* (medium communism), a "recommended" rating.

Perhaps after logging countless entries of *Putt-Putt* and *Freddi Fish* games, the authors noted that the titles that met their "recommended" standard were not, in fact, wholehearted endorsements, or even recommendations at all. Rather, they were simply *leftovers*—games that were outdated, mostly for children, and no longer relevant to today's audiences. (I personally could not find a single *Pajama Sam* Twitch stream, at least). They had to fudge their own recommendation standards to include "cool" games.

Like every censorship effort of the past, the "curators" had curated themselves into the most boring, irrelevant corner. After flagging 1,145 titles for "woke" content, the only games they had left to recommend *just weren't cool*, and when you're a self-appointed tastemaker and cultural authority, recommending something that just isn't that fun hurts your credibility. Their selections could never compete with the popularity and cultural gravitas of games they raged against as too "woke," such as *Baldur's Gate 3*. And this is what always happens with censorship efforts: The point is rage and domination. By cutting out anything that challenges their worldview, they arrive at their own dullness, and make everything they hate all the more desirable.

The things rage loves are boring; if games teach us anything, it's that life blooms in defiance.

//

These days, fantasy role-playing video games are my only luxury. The role-play is consuming, soothing, numbing, and the only way I know how to regulate my nervous system and get myself out of overwhelm and functional freeze in a state of constant social urgency. This is a small comfort I feel tremendous guilt about. I am forty-two years old and have somehow ended up in a world I don't recognize, engulfed in flame, paid for by my tax dollars. I have stumbled painfully through a doctorate only to be blindsided by divorce; I have $92K in student loan debt and feel bound by an uncertain future—*Is that job in a sanctuary state? Will my parents be deported? Will I lose my citizenship?* I donate to a family in Gaza's GoFundMe; donate to a friend's mutual aid fund for rent. "We're all counting on you!" my brother jokes. Can I even count on myself? Reality is unbearable; I need to know another world is possible.

I know what you're thinking: *Escapism is not how you change the world.* And you're right. But I'm not sure what I'm doing is escapism. I bring all of my problems with me; grapple with what feels hard to access as I ask Lucanis to Abominate in a combo attack with me. "Beautiful, Rook!" he says with love and admiration. Fantasy is where I have the power to topple tyrants and change a burning world, where my actions can actually help people, where I can solve problems.

Where someone loves me.

Fantasy is a place where my brain is not trying to kill me. Monsters are; tyrants are; power-mad gods are, and I beat them.

It is where I grieve the lost parts of myself, and reconnect with them for a little while—the wife, the object of someone's desire, the friend, the fighter, the defender, the helper. It is where gender roles are not compulsory, where my fourteen-year-old self, rebelling against strict Mexican parents and *machista* gender roles, doesn't have to be a daughter, and my present self can take a break from the constant labors of motherhood for a little while.

Most problematically, playing as an elf is where I grieve the fantasy of reclaiming my indigeneity, of inhabiting a precolonial self that has not been severed by *mestizaje* and assimilation, and imagine reconnection—imagine the world before the ships. It is the only place left to imagine wholeness. Fantasy is a site of imagined memory; it is also a site of (im)possible futures.

The Veilguard was also the first time I could play as truly nonbinary, with they/them pronouns, unbound to typically gendered body types. Usually, I play as a beautiful female elf, but *not* white—brown skin, black hair, dark brown eyes—an idealized form, finally compliant with the beauty standards of my gender. But this time, I played her—them—as nonbinary, working out the deepest knots of dysphoria in a safe environment through role-play.

I could experience what that kind of embodiment felt like in the world without committing to a pronoun change. And in that vulnerability, a memory: I've known, without having the language, that I was nonbinary as early as fourth grade, and I identified as a "tomboy." Later, I expressed gender nonconformity in acts of rebellion throughout my adolescence, refusing the obedience of Mexican daughterhood, knowing it only led to the self-denial of Mexican womanhood. I tried to look and sound like Kurt Cobain, and was heavily punished and pathologized as crazy for it. And when queerness and gender nonconformity become attached to "crazy," assimilation to cisheterosexuality is survival. Assimilation means you're sane. A deep conditioning took over and executed the program of "womanhood" into the rest of my life.

If I were young now, I'd have time to establish my identity as nonbinary and finally have the language for what I am. But to take it on now? I feel like I'm too old to start over. I have lived this life as a woman, and failed at it—beauty, marriage, mother-hood. I have endured its violences, known racism and misogyny twisted so tightly together that it's hard to untangle them now. I can't let that part of my identity, my history, and its pronoun go. Not now, at least. Perhaps it is a kind of self-denial—*I don't want my kid to have to call me "they" at school, I don't want to annoy his dad, I don't want to raise red flags with our custody agreement, I don't want to annoy or alienate my immigrant parents.* The anchors of my world keep me in *she*; but in Thedas, I can be *them*.

Asmongold, and everyone who tried to claim that having trans and nonbinary gender options in *The Veilguard* "forced people to be trans" were wrong. I had the opposite experience. *The Veilguard*, by creating the possibility for different expressions of gender, through role-playing as nonbinary, helped me make peace with being cis, and the kid within me too. In the space the game offers to experience nonbinary embodiment, I arrived at she/her. She/they.

My kid, on the other hand, is questioning their gender iden-tity. At my house, and in the imaginative space of their drawings, they write that they are nonbinary and use they/them pronouns. Sometimes they go back to he/him. They're not allowed to use they/them pronouns at their dad's house; he says our kid is too young to understand what that is. We mostly use he pronouns, out of habit, until they see me, their mom, playing a nonbinary character. *Oh! Your character is nonbinary, like me!* They are in fourth grade. I follow their lead, use whatever pronoun they want—in a family structure where they have to go by "he" at their dad's house, but can try on any pronoun at my house, games are just another space of affirmation.

I'M STILL LEARNING

MISS PEPPERMINT

I've found who I am, and it comes from the
Black women who came before me.

Do you know the feeling of waking up from a nightmare, realizing that you are safe, at home, in bed? I think we've all experienced that at one time or another. We take notice of the fear we feel, paying attention to how it moves through our body: the tension, the temperature, the quickness of breath, all of which comes from our instinct to fight or to flee. This is how I felt when I had a sudden Awakening about the United States, the Western world, and my place in it. The irony is that I felt like I had woken up from a nightmare and I was safe, but in actuality I was waking from peace and falling into a nightmare. This doesn't mean I'm not enormously grateful for everyone I've met, the connections that I've made, the experiences that I've had, the things that I've learned, the people that I've loved, the flavors that I've tasted, the memories that I've made, the achievements that I have been recognized for, and the efforts that I haven't been recognized for. I'm grateful for all of it. All of it makes me who I am and, more important, shapes who I will become.

For so long I had a very simplistic view of how the world worked, how society interacted, and how people like me fit into it. I knew that I'd been born and assigned male gender at birth. I knew I was expected to do things that boys did. I also knew that I was obviously queer because I was reminded of it every day by everyone around me. I knew that we were poor and that my family valued education; I knew I was a disappointment in that regard. I knew that I was Black. I was also acutely aware that my Blackness meant hundreds of years of having been targeted and discriminated against, and because of it, I would be treated as "less than" in certain situations.

Despite knowing all of that, I was very grateful to have been born when I was, because I knew I'd been born into a time that would allow me to escape all of those things—at least to a certain extent.

//

Growing up in a Black, single-parent household, surrounded by women, meant a strong relationship with my mother. Ours resembled friendship more than a traditional mother-daughter relationship. I was bullied for being queer and teased for the way I spoke even though it was the only way I knew how to speak. Some people in my community accused me of "talking white," another thing that set me apart and also drew attention toward me. I didn't know a lot of out queer kids growing up, either, so in many ways it was just my mother and I.

Being raised by her, and surrounded by Black women, I never felt out of place when my family was around. But in other kinds of spaces—social and community settings like school or church—the combination of my Blackness and queerness kept me ostracized. I was too white, even though I'm not white at all, and in many settings my Blackness felt hypervisible because I was so often the only Black person in the room. My mother and the Black women around me were always my safe haven.

For so many years, Black women have been labeled uneducated and treated as "less than" due to discrimination. But it was these Black women who formed me, who taught me to use my voice and how to speak, and who guided me when I experienced prejudice and racism along my journey. My family was highly educated, and everything about them reflected that education because we felt it was something to be proud of. As a kid, I was proud of the way I spoke because it reflected this, and I felt that my vocabulary and vernacular might have made me more relatable to white people than I otherwise would've been.

//

One of the women I was surrounded by in childhood was my grandmother. She helped to raise me, which means that we spent a lot of time together. I watched her interact with all kinds of women—in settings from the beauty parlor to the grocery store to the post office. So often the world required her to smash the low expectations people had for her, expectations that came from nothing more than their assumptions about her because of her being a Black woman of a certain age. There was a real dichotomy between her—a Black woman who was highly educated—and the white women she dealt with who worked in retail. I grew up seeing a strong sense of togetherness among Black women and femmes—an ability to coexist and relate to one another, and the camaraderie and community that grows from that—which often isn't understood by those outside the bounds of that community. I have rarely, if ever, seen that same camaraderie among women across racial lines.

When I was a young student in school, teachers always told my mother that I was extremely talkative and very well dressed. I don't look back at my life from that age and consider myself stylish, mostly because I was so young, and because my gender expression was that of a boy. But I did what I could, and as a seven- or eight-year-old, that meant dressing up for school in my Sunday best—dress clothes! We're talking three-piece suits, slacks, button-down shirts, and dress shoes. It didn't matter the weather, season, or activity. Dressing well felt like a form of protection, one way I could show the world who I truly was.

My taste was reinforced by some of the cultural icons I loved, then and now: Prince, MC Hammer, and Janet Jackson. They were wearing zoot suits and pinstripes, straight out of a Dick Tracy comic book. The style in the early '90s was buttoned up and dressed up, for sure. What I wore to school was simply my own flavor.

In those days my grandmother made a lot of my clothing, but one day she took me to purchase a suit for a special family occasion. It was going to be hand-tailored in the store. When we walked in, a slightly older-looking white woman who worked there barely acknowledged us, and the glances she did throw our way were patronizing, at best. I remember most the curious smirk on her face, as if what she really wanted to say was that our questions didn't matter because we couldn't even afford to be in that store. Every time she spoke, it seemed that each reply grew snarkier than the last. This was in stark comparison to the jovial and accommodating approach she took with the other shopper in the store, who—notably—was not Black. You can imagine how easy it was to come to the conclusion that we weren't wanted in that store, that we had not been, and never would be, welcome.

I felt deflated, was somehow embarrassed that my grandmother was being treated this way. I bore witness to her seemingly irrevocable power as it was dissolved before my eyes. The woman who worked in the store did tend to us, eventually, as was her job. But she rushed through it, bringing us the wrong size while my grandmother politely suggested ways to alter the suit so it would fit me properly. The woman refused to listen. And while I tried my best to pay attention, I was young, imaginative, prone to flights of fancy and daydreaming. I was in my own world, so it shocked me when I heard my grandmother raise her voice to this (white!) stranger, in my defense. She accused the woman of treating us unfairly, and then said something I'll never forget: "I will buy and sell your ass!"

I remember that as vividly as the day I first heard it. It was in that moment that I realized that my grandmother, who was not only college educated but an educator herself—and a very accomplished woman in her own right—was not a woman to allow herself to be disrespected, even by someone who carried social capital and support. Years later I learned that she had led boycotts of anti-Black businesses around the city and was very successful in her efforts. I don't even remember what happened with the suit that day; that's not part of the story. What I'm getting at is the specific sense of pride, self-determination, and self-confidence that my grandmother instilled in me, alongside the rest of my family. This is the legacy I'm reminded of when people ask me how I'm so happy and confident in my own skin. Of course I deal with insecurities, the same as anybody else, but I've always been able to see the brighter side. I've always had and expressed gratitude, which I think has saved me from spiraling into self-doubt and the crippling fear of scarcity, two things I believe are an entertainer's worst enemies.

Most of my experiences were shaped by the women I watched around me and on film, on television, and in music. There were very few pop culture references in film and television that dared to portray a Black queer femme person, and when they did, that person was often the butt of the joke. I looked instead to the women around me, saw my reflection in their intelligence and strength, and that sustained me. As I grew up I was able to recognize the very clear and very strong, yet unspoken, connection between Black cis women and queer femmes. Perhaps it was because those cis women bore witness to the type of treatment that Black trans women and queer femmes were often subjected to by the cishet men around them. Often, it was treatment that was in alignment with what these women received themselves. It seemed there was an induction into The Sisterhood, even though the alliance was unofficial. I would like to think that even if my grandmother hadn't been present that day, any Black woman witnessing me would've seen me for who I was, seen me being poked and prodded and talked down to, and would've snatched up that white sales attendant and stepped in, offering a motherly sort of protection.

These days, the story seems completely different. The built-in sisterhood and automatic understanding is still there, but that familiarity is weaponized against those of us who carry the least power and social capital within the sisterhood. There seems to be a built-in resentment, almost as if a traumatic experience is about to repeat itself. This might be caused by the impact of AIDS on the Black community and the demonizing of gay Black men who were forced to remain in the closet, sneaking around.

The white women who revel in the exclusion and suppression of trans women seem to view us as a physical threat. They cite a fear of being sexualized by men who pose as trans women to gain access to their safe, female-only spaces for the express purpose of harming women. I see this as a performative affirmation that young white women and girls remain in constant and inherent danger. It serves the false narrative that trans women and people of color are inherently dangerous, and that white women and girls must rely on protection from powerful men to remain safe. In villainizing trans women, and in particular trans women of color, white women put a target on the backs of all trans women—and many cis women who don't conform to traditional gendered expectations—while simultaneously ceding their power to men in hopes of remaining protected. My impression is that many white women defend the patriarchy by modeling how women should look and act, while shifting accountability for sexual assault from male attackers to trans women.

There is also a particular type of trans misogynoir that allows some Black women to view trans women as competition. Those women fear that they will lose the men they love to a trans woman. Time and time again, we see online conversations where cis Black women express fear, anger, and resentment at the possibility of being replaced by trans women. They say, repeatedly, with their chests, that trans women will *never* have what cis Black women have.

And here is, perhaps, the most interesting of intersections: cis Black women who see trans women as a threat and feel the need to exert power over them, uphold the patriarchy by shifting accountability for infidelity from their own husbands and sexual partners to trans women. The men can't be to blame if trans women are tricking the men into loving, or at least, desiring them. This absolves men of their own desire and turns trans women into the ultimate "other woman."

Either way, trans women—and especially Black trans women and femmes—are used as a scapegoat to pay the price of harmful behavior that men have historically perpetrated on women. This is especially true when you consider the many violent—and often improperly investigated and prosecuted—assaults and murders perpetrated against trans women by our intimate partners: our lovers and sometimes even our boyfriends.

Ironically, trans men are typically and almost exclusively left out of this conversation.

//

As a young person I struggled to figure out exactly how to fit in, how to make and have friends. I wasn't terribly good at it, but that loneliness really helped me discover my purpose and the drive I needed to be excellent in that purpose. From a young age, I yearned to understand my purpose, because I knew that the typical heteronormative life—a house with a white picket fence and two kids in the yard—wasn't my jam. Instead, I saw community, chosen family, and drag entertainment—with a twist. Also, I was a product of the '90s MTV era, when every celebrity on the red carpet wore a red AIDS ribbon and the biggest divas were rocking the vote; it felt like the real world was breaking LGBTQ boundaries. I loved and looked up to Rickie from *My So-Called Life* and Pedro Zamora from *The Real World*. I knew that a sense of activism was going to be baked into whatever path life led me down.

These are the types of moments that led me to the set of *Pose*, where I was able to witness Black trans performers, many of whom were on a professional filming set for the first time. Certainly there must have been at least one person who was spared, at least for one day, from engaging in survival sex work. It's ironic, given the job discrimination and disproportionate murder rate of Black trans women at the hands of intimate partners, that such work often proves so dangerous and even deadly.

Even advocating for yourself, for your community, and for the rights of others can be dangerous, especially when you're on the front lines of protest. Black women and femmes have been at the front lines of virtually every social justice movement that I've been able to participate in. I take pride in that, but I also recognize the risk involved.

Stories like those of Harriet Tubman and Ida B. Wells are inspiring, but they're so far in the past that they can sometimes feel like they're from another world. But when I think of my grandmother and what she instilled in me, I see a lineage of standing up for myself, for my community, and for those who need it. My obsession with using my platform and personal resources to advocate for our community is an extension of the legacies of folks like Marsha P. Johnson and William Dorsey Swann, the gender nonconformist who was put in prison for hosting balls and drag parties, and later petitioned the federal government for release. His petition became the first instance, on record, of LGBTQ+ rights being advocated for through the legal system. Whenever I have a moment of doubt, I think of and am grateful for people like Marsha and William, both of whom I consider my ancestors—or my transcestors.

It's these stories and histories, paired with my own experiences, that help me feel well equipped to navigate through life as a performer and entertainer while using my platform to speak out for every cause that's important to me. Whether it be arranging AIDS/HIV testing during my shows, donating money to local LGBTQ charities, marching across the Brooklyn Bridge for marriage equality, or raising money for pro-LGBTQ organizations, I feel like I've found my purpose, I've found who I am, and it comes from the Black women who came before me, who raised me, who ensured that I grew up with a social conscience.

One might say that I spend more time doing all of this than I do actually working as an actor. But I wouldn't change a second of it. I've learned some valuable lessons, and every day I'm still learning.

STRAINING TOWARD HUMANITY

TRANS WOMEN AS SAINT AND SHADOW

KAI CHENG THOM

Trans women and trans femmes occupy a locus
of extreme intensity in the cultural imagination.

In the dream, I am an enormous immortal transgender woman, some thirty or forty feet tall, who has fallen from the sky. Where my body strikes the earth, a crater forms and buildings topple, but wherever my glowing cerulean blood soaks into the soil, plant life blooms in profusion.

My limbs are broken, so I cannot move. The humans who live in the place where I have landed realize that my blood is a source of incredible power, and so they decide to worship me as a goddess, building a great and beautiful temple up around me. They insert pipelines into my body to siphon away my blood, to be used for a wide range of spiritual, medical, and industrial purposes.

//

It's been more than ten years since I transitioned, and it often seems to me that the world I live in has ended and begun anew several times in those years. Certainly the young Chinese girl I was at twenty-two, just starting to dream into the possibility of life as a woman, would be astounded by the life I lead today as a trans cultural worker and healer amid a veritable sea of trans peers.

That girl could not have imagined that her face would be one of many trans women's faces to appear on billboards for major fashion brands, or that the work of trans women of color celebrities such as Laverne Cox or the stars of the TV show *Pose* would reach millions of fans. She would not believe that the novel she was writing, nor the books of her transfeminine peers, would become bestsellers, win awards, find the readership of a generation of trans people as far as thousands of miles away.

Yet that girl would also not have imagined that in this same future, she would experience even more hatred and fear than she ever had before. She did not know that she and her transfeminine sisters would occupy the role of inspirational revolutionary figure and angelic martyr, simultaneously with the role of terrifying sexualized monster at the center of an inflamed social panic that continues to spread today.

Trans women and trans femmes occupy a locus of extreme intensity in the cultural imagination. Our bodies are a lightning rod for projection, a focal point through which the dominant culture offloads its latent anxieties and repressed longings about gender, sexuality, beauty, violence, freedom, and death. As a result, the specter of the trans woman is also a nexus for polarized archetypes within the cultural consciousness: We are always the saint yet always the shadow, always the martyr yet always the monster. We are always symbols and never people.

Even within the queer community and the putatively "social justice left," this dynamic of simultaneous pedestalization and demonization persists; the same community that speaks of transfem historical figures such as Marsha P. Johnson and Sylvia Rivera with breathless reverence and even burns votive candles inscribed with their likenesses is swift to accuse trans women and femmes of dangerous insanity and sexual predation. Trans woman writer Morgan M Page documents this phenomenon in her 2015 essay "Crazy Trans Woman Syndrome," as does Porpentine Charity Heartscape in her viral and controversial online piece "Hot Allostatic Load."

Simply put, the majority of people have strong feelings about us, often without really knowing why. When a trans woman or transfeminine person walks into a room and is perceived as trans (whether because she does not "pass" to those beholding her or because she intentionally comes out as such), she is met with awe, disgust, fear, desire. To the world, we are monsters in the sense of the Latin *monstrum*: living omens, breathing portents, embodied harbingers of ruin or rapture.

The transphobic hate campaigns intended to vilify our community and legislate us out of existence are most often centered around the image of the trans woman as a disgusting pervert lurking around the corner of every women's bathroom and women's shelter. Society is quick to ridicule those who express attraction to us. Yet "shemale" porn has been one of the most popular categories of pornography on the internet for decades.

Of course, these deeply divided reactions say very little about the personhood of trans women and quite a lot about the collective consciousness of the dominant culture. Namely, they speak to a psychosexual complex lurking at the heart of patriarchal gender and sexuality norms, the terror and yearning that burn in the heart of a society constructed around the veneration of a rigidly violent form of heterosexuality that robs men and women of their fullest humanity and erotic freedom.

Yet my concern in this essay is less about the meaning of the simultaneous pedestalization and demonization of trans women for broader society and more about its impact on the psyche of transfeminine people. What does it mean to be the constant recipients of such intense and fractured projections? What does carrying the burden of being the dominant culture's psychosexual scapegoat do to a body, a mind, a soul over time? Where does the spark of our humanity still shimmer, hidden amid all the smoke and mirrors?

//

In the dream, I am a huge transfeminine goddess shackled to an enormous altar in a place that is both my temple and my prison. The people come here to both worship and consume me; it is unclear where worship ends and consumption begins. It is unclear whether this is my punishment or my reward. The people might adore me, or perhaps they fear me. Regardless, the end is the same. I am eaten either way—or perhaps not. Perhaps I'm not ready.

I thrash about on the altar to which I am bound. I'm not sure how long I have waited, in patience, for the people to set me free. I'm not sure how long I've been trying to bear the weight of their needs, their fears, their hatred, their love. All I know is that it's been too long, and suddenly I am full of rage. The chains that hold me groan and shriek, but they can no longer bind me. They shatter, and as I tear free of the altar, I am transforming, shape-shifting, legs and arms elongating and multiplying, the joints of my limbs turning themselves inside out as my teeth lengthen and fuse into a set of mandibles large and strong enough to tear a human being in half.

Now I have eight terrible limbs on which to crawl like a gigantic spider and snapping, slavering jaws through which I hiss and snarl. The people all around me scream in terror, fleeing as quickly as they can, and I shake with cruel, jubilant laughter, drinking in their fear. *Yes, run away!* I call mockingly after them. *Run away, my devoted worshippers! Your goddess has fed you and now it is her turn to feast!*

//

In 2011, transfeminine Filipinx and multidisciplinary artist Mark Aguhar included the following words in her artwork *Not You (Power Circle)*, now immortalized among a certain cohort of queer and trans people of color: "WHO IS WORTH MY LOVE, MY STRENGTH & MY RAGE?" This defiant assertion of the artist's own worth and dignity exemplifies the central themes of Aguhar's work, which included a ferocious interrogation of racism, fatphobia, and the unrelenting dehumanization of brown transfeminine people within and outside of queer communities.

As a creator, Aguhar was known—and, among my own cohort of millennial queer and trans artists of color, renowned—for her unapologetic voice, her emotional range, and the vibrancy with which she gave life to our struggle to be seen as human, as well as her fierce refusal of any demand that she soften her tone in order to make herself more palatable to the white gaze, the white gays, or mainstream heterosexual culture.

Tragically, Aguhar died by suicide at the age of twenty-four in 2012, on March 12, in a terrible loss for her loved ones as well as for the transfeminine community. In an odd twist of fate that still troubles me at times, March 12 also happens to be my birthday.

Mark Aguhar's full-throated articulation of transfeminine rage echoes with the voices of many trans women and transfem activists, thinkers, and cultural workers of the past several decades who respond to the vilification of our existence by embracing the dominant culture's projection of its own shadow onto us. This instinctive collective strategy is about embracing the fearsome power of the archetypes of exile, outcast, angry activist, dangerous being, monster, and so on, that have been assigned to our bodies. In essence, it is about saying to oneself and the world, *So they fear me? Then let them fear me.*

Variations on this theme can be found across the spectrum of transfeminine cultural production, including in Susan Stryker's seminal 1994 essay, "My Words to Victor Frankenstein Above the Village of Chamounix," in which she declares, "I want to lay claim to the dark power of my monstrous identity . . . I am a transsexual, and therefore I am a monster." Stryker explicitly links "transsexual monstrosity" with "transgender rage," a link that remains a central curiosity within transfeminine cultural consciousness, if our literature and art are any indication.

Fantasist Maya Deane, for example, reimagines the mythological Achilles as a terrifying trans woman warrior in her novel *Wrath Goddess Sing*, while the aforementioned Porpentine Charity Heartscape envisions a world of enormous biomechanical warbeast mechas piloted by transfem fighters in *Psycho Nymph Exile*. Meanwhile, bestselling trans woman authors Torrey Peters and Gretchen Felker-Martin, in their respective works *Infect Your Friends and Loved Ones* and *Manhunt*, explore postapocalyptic worlds in which trans women are forced to engage in gruesome acts of violence in order to survive.

For many of us, embracing the shadow of the monster and the potency of our rage is often a portal to rediscovering our agency. By reclaiming the monstrous role assigned to us, and by embodying the rightful rage that comes with receiving such a role, we give ourselves both the permission and the power to use the fear and discomfort that the world projects onto us to push back against the restraints placed on our freedom.

Yet the question that still haunts me is this: Where does the reclamation of the archetypal monstrous (or monstress) trans woman end and my true personhood begin? Is there such a thing as "my true personhood" to begin with? If I lean too far into the shadow, is there a chance I'll never return?

//

In the dream, I am a giant immortal transgender woman who is adored and cherished by all. Ten thousand years ago, I fell from the sky and landed among the people here, who discovered that my blood had the power to heal their wounds and cure their diseases, while my body had the power to help their crops grow.

Though at first they were afraid and suspicious, I won their trust by selflessly giving of myself to meet their needs and soothe their fears. Wherever I encounter a wounded or sick person, I let them drink of my glowing cerulean blood, and they are healed. Whenever the crops fail, I bury a slice of my own flesh in the fields, and the food grows anew. I have learned that sacrifice and softness are the way of survival.

Yet my body grows weaker and weaker as the years go by. My arteries and veins are starting to run dry. I am tired, so tired. And each time I give of myself to assuage the hunger of the people who love me, I feel the light inside me—the light of the stars from which I came—fade a little more. Soon, I can sense, that light will go out forever and my flesh and blood will cease to yield their miraculous gifts. The people will grow afraid, and then angry, as they begin to succumb to diseases, as the weather turns and the harvest season is lean.

And then, I think, they will come for me.

//

The mirror image of the monstrous trans woman is the trans woman as sainted angel, a creature too good for this wicked world. Notably, it often seems more common that trans women and transfeminine individuals are elevated to this status posthumously, as is the case with literal saints. No doubt it is easier to find the dead faultless than the living, who are often inconveniently prone to committing fresh sins at any moment.

Marsha P. Johnson and Sylvia Rivera, legendary participants in and leaders of the Stonewall Uprising and founders of the Street Transvestite Action Revolutionaries (STAR) House in 1970, are often venerated within the queer and trans community—indeed, I venerate them myself, and I think rightly so, to a large extent. Yet I also cannot help but wonder about the extent to which the breathless adoration of these two human beings, and particularly the use of their names and images as part of a subcultural myth-making, flattens their memory and erases the texture of who they were in life.

Marsha P. Johnson was seventeen years old when she met Sylvia Rivera, who was eleven at the time, and they were approximately twenty-five and nineteen when they started the STAR House—a four-bedroom apartment with no heating or electricity in which they sheltered homeless queer youth and which they kept running with funds made through sex work. Let us imagine real people, real racialized transfeminine youth in these positions, and all the responsibility and chaos that undoubtedly came with them, rather than martyrs and saints. Let us imagine how real people might respond to those conditions.

It is well documented that Sylvia Rivera, at least, could be ferocious in demeanor when the spirit moved her. I like to think the same is true of Marsha P. Johnson. In my most blasphemous moments, I like to imagine that they both would be considered *problematic* by the standards of today's social justice movement—that they were "bad bitches," as the saying goes. I enjoy this blasphemous idea of them more than the image of Saint Sylvia and Saint Marsha because the blasphemous idea makes me feel closer to them.

Among the living, trans women and trans femmes are subjected to great pressure to live saintly lives as a precarious bid for survival in a world that fears and hates us. During the so-called Transgender Tipping Point years of the mid-2010s, the burden of this pressure was exemplified by the intense media attention placed upon transfeminine people, particularly cultural figures such as the iconic actress Laverne Cox, who responded to the scrutiny of those years with what can only be described as astounding grace and poise.

Cox has often spoken on and advocated for trans rights, integrating a sophisticated analysis of race, class, and other aspects of social justice while doing so. Cox's positive impact on society cannot be understated. I wonder, however, about the toll her public-facing role may have taken on her spirit and what violences she may have experienced as a Black trans woman in a deeply anti-Black and transmisogynist cultural landscape.

In an interview on the television show *Totally Biased with W. Kamau Bell*, Cox coined the term *possibility model* as an alternative to *role model* to describe her desired impact on society. She suggests that a possibility model is someone whose public persona inspires others to live their dreams despite repressive and oppressive social norms. The idea is poignant. Yet I cannot help but long for a world in which queer and trans people do not lack so desperately for possibility—and in which trans women are not so often called upon to provide it at the cost of our own complexity.

//

Sometimes when I wake up in the mornings, I'm afraid to leave my home. This is a feeling that the girl I used to be knew well, but the woman I am today is always surprised when the anxiety suddenly appears like a ghost I thought I'd left behind. I've done so many things, been so many places, since coming out as trans. Yet the fear still lives somewhere deep inside my body.

There was a time when I used to wear ripped denim and sequined vests to go outside, and shimmering makeup with an asymmetrical haircut. I was a glam punk gender bender, a performance artist who tore her own skin open with her fingernails onstage to prove a point: That I feared nothing. That I was ferocious, a fierce femme, a creature of the shadows and the glittering night. I wrote a book about a trans girl gang that hunts and beats up straight men for fun. I had to write it quickly, before I turned twenty-five, because I didn't believe I would live much longer than that.

Nowadays, I wear a lot of business casual, yoga clothes, and sensible shoes. I am a wellness influencer on the internet, and my branding is all about love. I have had emails from people all over the world telling me what an inspiration I am. I have spoken to crowded rooms to rapt attention. Yet when I step out onto the street, I never know what will happen, how I will be received.

I am a person who is stared at; I have been for my entire adult life, no matter what I wear. I am a mirror to others of what they yearn and fear to be. Sometimes, parents pull their children closer when I am near. Sometimes, a straight-looking father with a toddler in tow will stare at me with hunger in his eyes. Sometimes I hate that and sometimes I enjoy it. I am the devourer. I am the devoured. I wish I could disappear. Let them stare. Once, a woman stopped me in the subway to tell me that I was the most beautiful person she'd ever seen.

Then there are moments when none of it matters: When I am walking in the summer sunlight, or when the autumn wind is strong and there are leaves in my hair, or when I am by the lake beneath the stars. When I am in the arms of particular lovers who hold me in a particular way, whispering my name. In those moments, I am neither saint nor shadow, neither monster nor martyr, but simply spirit made flesh, longing given life. I have touched completeness, which is to say miraculous imperfection. I am nothing and no one except myself.

FEMININITY WAS THE KNIFE I WIELDED

JONAH WU

Masculinity was the soft and
vulnerable thing inside me.

At the clinic, my RN patiently explains to me how to change the eighteen-gauge needle to the thinner twenty-five-gauge, how to swab the side of my thigh with an alcohol wipe to prep it for injection. I can barely hear him; my head feels like it's underwater, and my hands are shaking. When I push the air bubbles out of the syringe and the excess fluid dribbles down along the needle's length, my RN nods at me. "Whenever you're ready," he says, softly, as if not to startle me.

"And it just goes in—all at once?" I ask, even though we've already gone over this once before.

"If you can," he confirms. "It'll hurt less, that way."

In this moment, poking myself with a needle for the first time feels impossible. I am terrified of needles. Through the haze of my anxiety, I briefly consider that this is an apt metaphor for my decision to take testosterone—that I was the one who chose to do this, that it is not the act itself but the unknowability of the result that I am most fearful of, but also that it is impossible to waver any longer. I am on the precipice; the syringe is already in my hand, poised in its perpendicular position, ready to pierce through my thigh and all of my jittery nerves.

My hand stills. At last, I'm ready. It's time to take the plunge.

//

At some point last year, my Instagram algorithm finally figured out that I am a queer guy. Not a difficult task, as I had been clicking on every suggested Reel of a hot Asian man, half out of a desire to study and steal what made them so effortlessly masculine, and half out of *desire*. It spat out video after video for me of men in slo-mo or match-cut transitions, flaunting their perfectly styled hair and expensive outfits, and like a particularly naive mark, I watched them all. But there were a couple of Reels mixed in with the rest that took me aback. Catching sight of a blond-haired Japanese man dressed up in gallant period attire, poised and tall under a spotlight and singing his heart out onstage, I knew from previous experience that he was not a man at all, but Rei Yuzuka, formerly one of the top stars of Japan's Takarazuka Revue, an all-female theater troupe. Yuzuka is an *otokoyaku*—a (presumably) cis female performer who plays only men's roles, and she is the best among a notoriously competitive company of actresses. It did not escape my notice, either, that Yuzuka had managed to fool my Instagram algorithm—that, with the sheer power of her gender performance, she had transed my panoptic gaze just a little bit.

"Part of the especially unique allure of the Takarazuka Revue," the official YouTube channel boasts, "is how the women playing otokoyaku seem to be more impressive on stage than real men." Which is a statement that, as a transmasculine person, I find incredibly funny. Because isn't that, in effect, what I am doing? Constructing an alluring masculine fantasy for myself, out of the bits and pieces I observed and borrowed from other men? Like the otokoyaku, I wasn't always a man. I had to learn to become one.

//

I hadn't always wanted to be transmasculine. At the beginning of 2018, with the help of my therapist and several close friends, I left my boyfriend. It had been a physically and emotionally abusive relationship, punctuated by several instances of sexual assault, and I had settled into my new apartment, away from him, somewhat shattered as a person.

It had unequivocally been a relationship filled with gendered violence, despite his protestations that he was a feminist, just because of the way cisheteronormativity shutters us into gendered roles if we don't actively resist it. Knowing this, and filled with a redolent rage at what he had done to me, I couldn't help but feel vengeful. This was, perhaps, at the height of the "men are trash" rhetoric spreading around social media, with everyone happily tweeting and sharing easy zingers. Including me. It felt righteous and justified, and moreover, in my injured psyche, it made sense. Masculinity had hurt me, which meant that I had to take shelter from it. I imagined that femininity was a divine goodness. Masculinity was something toxic to be rooted out in everyone and destroyed. I held on to this belief for several years, especially since it was a sentiment echoed in many queer spaces that I had called my community.

And yet, in 2021, I suddenly felt like I wanted to go on testosterone.

//

The way I have described it to my friends is that my body knew before my mind did. By 2021, I had already come out as nonbinary, changed my name to Jonah on all fronts but the legal one, and even started presenting as more masculine, but I had never thought that I would want to undergo medical transition or to be seen as, first and foremost, a man. I still can't fully explain how I knew it was testosterone that my body needed, and not anything else. All I can really say is that it was a visceral urge that seemed to spring from some deeper part of me that came before language and reason.

These urges came on the heels of my abruptly quitting a longtime job, and I don't think the timing was pure coincidence. Freed from the last stranglehold that required me to put on a pretense for polite society, I was suddenly thrust into discovering who I was outside of professionalism and capitalism for the first time in three years. But the thought of wanting to go on T was terrifying. I couldn't understand it at the time: Why did I want to be a man, when men had hurt me so much?

There is a lot of fearmongering about testosterone and how it affects one's emotions, mostly designed to dissuade trans men from transitioning and to give cis men a biological excuse for their harmful behavior. The fearmongering is so pervasive on every level of society that it's hardly questioned, and I certainly believed a lot of it when I first began researching what it would be like to go on T.

Like many others, the first things I learned about hormone replacement therapy (HRT) were largely from hearsay and haphazard Google searches. There seemed to be agreement that the effects of T were "destructive," "irreversible." You wouldn't be able to undo the rapid proliferation of facial and body hair, nor the deepened vocal cords, nor the bottom growth. Worst of all was the oft-discussed "roid rage," which made T sound like a poison that was destined to incur anger and aggression in any body it entered. That made me most afraid of testosterone—afraid that I would change too much as a person, afraid that I wouldn't recognize who I was in the mirror. What if T transformed me into the thing I feared most—a man who causes harm to other people?

It was this language that made me put off going on T for almost a whole year, all while I was in severe dysphoric pain. Fortunately, I was surrounded by good people—trans/nonbinary friends who graciously listened as I voiced my wants and worries, and specifically, a few transmasculine friends who were going through a similar process of discovery with their own genders. Through them, I learned that masculinity wasn't anything to feel ashamed of, and so was emboldened to try looking into HRT once again. I scoured Twitter for personal experiences from transmasc folks, I read crowdsourced Google Docs on the effects of T, and I watched YouTube videos and TikToks of trans guys talking about their transitions. This new variety of first-person reportage was invaluable to me; it showed me that there were many ways to be a man and to exist in a man's body with joy. Moreover, it taught me that the fearmongering was a result of TERF rhetoric, which sought to "preserve" and "protect" the femininity of transmasc folks and prevent them from transitioning.

I had femininity within me, certainly, but I didn't want it to define me anymore. If anything was poisoning me, it was the mantle of womanhood that was forced on me but that I had never wanted. And if I didn't remove it from myself, it might end up killing me. Slowly, my need drowned out my fear, and I gathered the courage to call my local gender clinic for an intake appointment. After years of enduring violence, I owed my body the chance at freedom and autonomy.

//

We do a lot of harm to ourselves and to others when we assume the bioessentialist stance that men, particularly cis men, are not capable of emotional intimacy. I remember receiving a verbal dressing down from an old friend when I called them complaining about the lack of investment I was getting from a guy in my burgeoning friendship with him. "You need more female friends," they told me. "Guys just aren't good at having deep heart-to-hearts." "But," I replied hesitantly, "I feel like I just get along better with men?" There are exceptions, of course, but I have often felt a sense of disconnect when befriending women—a gap of difference I never felt like I could bridge. "You're probably hanging on to some internalized misogyny" was my friend's diagnosis. "I think you have to ask yourself why female friends aren't good enough for you." Funnily enough, my friend would probably be horrified to be reminded that they once said such a thing to me. At the time, we both identified as cis women, and now neither of us does.

I had no good explanation for *why* I yearned for the emotional intimacy of men. Sometimes there is no logic devised for feelings; they are simply that: feelings—gestures toward an emotional truth that has no container. In Sophia Giovannitti's essay "In Defense of Men," a critique of the common liberal feminist impulse for man-hating, she writes, "I love men's casual homoerotic acknowledgments of each other *as men*; I want all men to kiss their homies goodnight and I want it so badly that I, too, want to be a man who is a homie who gets kissed goodnight." Giovannitti wrote this as a cishet woman, but I can find no better line to encapsulate my entire spectrum of *desire* as a queer trans guy. We all talk about how toxic cispatriarchal standards render many men isolated and unequipped to express intimacy. While that's certainly true, I have met many men (cis, trans, and nonbinary alike) who happily resist those values and are openly affectionate with their male friends, and when it happens, it is just as beautiful, sacred, and deserving of protection as any other expression of friendship.

I have no better proof of this than my own experience. Recently, a cis female friend who'd also experienced intimate partner violence asked me, "How did you stop yourself from blaming men as a whole for your trauma, and from going down the man-hating path?"

"I don't know," I confessed. "I guess I was just lucky to have some really good guy friends at the time."

In retrospect, I think it's funny that some of my most toxic, emotionally taxing friendships have been with queer femmes, and some of my most loving, intimate friendships have been with cishet men. Of course, I could say the exact opposite is true as well. The devastation of my twenties was caused by a man with whom

I was in a cishet-fronting relationship, and the people most responsible for rescuing me from it were women. I have been held and loved by people of all genders, and I have been hurt by them, too. Knowing we are all capable of harm regardless of our identity markers—that was ultimately the truth that freed me.

//

Where does that leave me, then? I want to acknowledge that a toxic masculinity does exist—one upheld by a cispatriarchal system that seeks to control and poison all of us, including cis men. I want to confirm that there is a power pageantry at play here that, if we're not careful, even transmasculine folks can be lured to participate in. And I want to emphasize that this model of masculinity is inextricable from the project of white supremacy, which stations its imagery of "ideal maleness" and "ideal femaleness" in white bodies and traditions. For Asians in particular, we are always feminized by the white gaze, regardless of gender. Even if I were attempting to "transition into male privilege," as some TERFs claim, it would never be possible for me. I am forever in America, by nature of my race and assigned sex at birth, designated to be some bastardized form of "gender," not the "desirable feminine," but certainly not masculine, either. So I don't belong in the traditional dichotomy of masculinity and femininity, and I don't care to, either.

Aligning masculinity with "hardness" and femininity with "softness" simply reifies gender binaries, the same way that primarily referring to nonbinary people as assigned female at birth (AFAB) or assigned male at birth (AMAB) does. Our social conditioning trains us to think in binaries, and it's a hard system to escape, even as our own genders manage to. On a practical level, I don't think these dichotomies make a whole lot of sense, either. Growing up, I was a rebellious and rambunctious tomboy, and my mother had (without much success) attempted to eradicate my inherent boyishness and impose femininity on me—not because she wanted femininity to make me soft, but because she thought my unacceptable gender deviance, which was out of alignment with the society I lived in, was my weakness. Possibly my worst offense to her was that I was a sensitive child, prone to crying and large emotions. She wanted me to hide that as well, under the clean and equanimous guise of a "good girl." "Never show the world your true face" was the lesson she stressed the most: "The smartest way to survive is to wear the face that everyone else wants to see."

Unthinkingly, I had swallowed her teachings, even when they had hurt me. All throughout my teens and early twenties, I taught myself how to perfect femininity. I spent years curating my wardrobe and took pride in being complimented for my style. This only intensified after I left my ex. In the typical post-breakup fashion, I wanted to prove that he hadn't hurt me at all, that I was stronger and better without him. I dyed my hair, bought more revealing clothes, and hunted for the gazes and praise that would affirm that I was worth their love. I'd even hazard to say that these attempts at high femme appearance were extremely successful. But one afternoon, returning from a party for which I had dressed to the nines, I walked back to my apartment feeling like I wanted to cry. Nothing bad had happened there; everyone had been perfectly nice to me. But I felt like the underside of my flesh was crawling, like I wanted to rip all of my skin off. And I knew precisely the source of my deep discomfort, even as I clung onto it, thinking it would save me.

To me, femininity was the knife I wielded, as well as my armor. Masculinity was the soft and vulnerable thing inside me that I had to protect from the cruelty of the world, that opened me up to the possibility of violence. For too long, I thought that this was the way it had to be. But as any person, cis or trans, might be able to tell you, this is a painful way of living. And it isn't even effective at saving you from harm. Lately, I have been discovering that a weaponless existence is the only way I know how to continue to live. Being free, weightless, and true to myself returns to me an innate strength that was hindered by the pressure to conform, and it also allows me to surround myself with people who are interested in loving me as whoever I am, no matter how many changes I may go through over time. I had been taught my whole life that being soft and vulnerable would only make me a sucker, a fool. But these days, I am finding that it is quite the opposite— that if I open up and meet people halfway, more often than not, they will come to meet me where I am.

//

I am lucky, in some ways, that the first trans man I encountered in any piece of fictional media was Oshima in Haruki Murakami's *Kafka on the Shore*. Fifteen years after I'd first read it, I now have some issues with how Oshima is depicted as well as the contents of the book itself, but Oshima is still very meaningful to me. His gender identity is never questioned by the other two main characters, and he occupies a position of wisdom and culture in the narrative that feels enviable. Anytime the titular teenager Kafka needs advice from a sensible mentor figure, Oshima is there to provide him with it, and anytime Murakami needs to deliver an excessively long monologue about his opinions of art, it comes out of Oshima's witty and discerning mouth. In a story with deliberately murky plotlines and morals, Oshima is the lighthouse, a beacon of warmth and stability that others can turn to when lost.

Moreover, Oshima runs completely counter to everything my mother wanted me to do: He invites strangers in need into his home without question, he is kind, he speaks his mind, and he doesn't care what others think. He can survive the world as himself; he doesn't need any armor. For years, Oshima was my favorite and most memorable part of *Kafka on the Shore*, and I didn't realize until recently that he represents a beacon for me, too, one that I can look back to and orient myself toward whenever I doubt that my masculinity is "enough." When I try conceiving of a gentle but strong transmasculinity, often I am remembering meeting Oshima for the first time on the page, in equal parts awe and envy.

I am thinking of him the first time I plunge the needle into my thigh—not just Oshima, but the person that I want to become, the person I have always suspected that I might actually be. My RN was wrong—the injection *still* hurts, but it actually doesn't hurt as much as I'd thought it would. Which is also an apt metaphor for my experience with testosterone. Now that it's been a few years on T for me, I'm finding that a lot of the commonly repeated things about T are, perhaps, not as common after all. Because of the haphazard game of genetics, there truly is no universal transition experience. My face and body have visibly changed, but not as quickly or drastically as everybody, even the most well-meaning of folks, would have led me to believe. And that, for the moment, is okay with me. I am gradually molting into the shape of my soul, which I can now see whenever I look in the mirror. I am not waking up to suddenly discover that I am a completely different person; I'm growing with myself, one day at a time.

More important, of course, is the way that I've been feeling on T. Counter to the prevalent myths, I don't feel out of control or particularly short-tempered, but rather more open and in touch with my emotions. For many years, I had put up so many walls, with others and with myself. I refused to let myself feel the totality of my feelings, convinced that the depth of them would destroy me. I'm realizing now that what felt so unmanageable was the fog of dysphoria that lay heavily over everything, making it challenging to face my most difficult issues or even to ascertain what their root causes were. With the dysphoria largely cleared away, it's like I'm reexperiencing myself in full color. Still capable of deep sorrow, yes, but not terrified that I'll be ruined in its wake. What's more, I possess a broader range of joy that makes me feel fully human, fully present and participating in the world around me. And that, to me, is what it means to be(come) a man.

The wonderful thing about being trans is that sometimes you discover the person you needed to become was always simply who you are. After years of wandering, I have finally come home to myself. There in my bones still lives the child who cries easily and bruises quickly, who gravitates toward warmth too readily but moves toward the fire without fear. I recognized him at once. Excavating them from buried earth, I take their hand in mine. I find that I no longer require the armor to live, to feel safe. After all, I am not walking forward alone, but with every part of myself.

THE GODDESS IN THE VOLCANO

GABRIELLE BELLOT

She was, in short, a vision of the kind of
unconstrained woman I wished to be.

The way to the volcano is a particular kind of dark, the sort of nightblack that feels palpable, heavy, filled with myths. In the beams of our rental car's headlights you can faintly see mist-drops of rain, remnants of a wandering storm from earlier that day. The sky is clearer now, though bulbous clouds drift in it like the sails of great ships, the occasional star visible between their puffs. The streetlamps along the tree-lined road are dim, their yellow glow like fireflies frozen in the air. The road is lonely, but we know the traffic will thicken as we get nearer to a viewing spot.

My wife and I are at Kīlauea in the Big Island in Hawaii, just a day after arriving for an anniversary trip, and we're in search of lava. I'm both excited and nervous. It's an unexpected quest to be on, in part because until we landed in Hawaii twenty-four hours earlier, we hadn't realized that the legendary volcano was active.

We'd woven together grand plans for our trip—a night dive with manta rays; a journey to the sacred peak of Mauna Kea to watch the sunset from above the clouds; an open-ocean snorkeling expedition to hopefully find sharks, dolphins, or whales to swim with; hiking; and, of course, relaxing—and we had been checking the lava forecasts. But Pele—the beautiful and terrible goddess of volcanoes in Hawaiian mythos, who created the Hawaiian Islands and still resides in Kīlauea—had been asleep until we arrived. Now, though, she was blinking back awake, and, like moths to a great flame, we'd been drawn to the fatal promise of her orangedark.

And drawn we are. My wife had never seen lava and told me as we planned our anniversary how much she hoped we would. I had been luckier. Many years earlier, I had seen lava once, though just for a few seconds. It was on a trip with my parents to the Big Island when I was a child. My parents had booked a helicopter tour, which involved flying along one coast of the island under the metallic drone of the propeller; at one point, I remember seeing a plume of smoke billowing into the air in front of us near a cliffside, for a trickle of lava, the pilot yelled over the din, was pouring into the sea. I couldn't see it through the smoke, though, and felt disappointed. Then, just as we were about to turn around, I glimpsed a bright, bold orange through the fumes, a fire-river gushing as if in slow motion.

It was only for a moment, but I always remembered that glimpse. There was something about it—but what that something was I couldn't have told you back then. It just touched something subterranean in me, like finding a candle lit in a cavern I'd never known was there, seen only by its distant glow.

Despite growing up myself on a volcanic island in the Caribbean, I've long felt closer to water—if I have to choose one of the classical elements. Although as a child I was scared of the oceans, imagining that the tentacles of great squids from the lightless depths were waiting to grab my ankles if I waded in too far or that the moment I let my feet touch the bottom I would step on the toxic barb of a stingray, I've always had a kinship with water, with its shades of blue. It's the imagery that always comes to me first when writing or self-describing: flows, waves, ripples, the blue of the sea, coral reefs, the elfin dance of light underwater, petrichor, the sound of heavy rain dense and august as some ancient cathedral. I love, too, the idea of water as a flexible, adaptable thing, able to be powerful as a maelstrom yet tending toward stillness and coolness.

As a quiet, melancholic introvert, the qualities of water and the resonances of the color blue more broadly just seem *right*.

Fire, by contrast, never seemed to fit someone like me, or so I thought. It seemed an element of extroversion, extirpation, eruptions of energy, an element for those comfortable standing out in a crowd. I like all of these qualities in theory but don't feel able to embody them.

And, as a queer kid in the closet who was often bullied for my temporary stammer, the odd timbre of my voice, and my general awkwardness, I didn't *want* to stand out. More often than not, I just wanted to disappear into some azure pool inside the earth, hidden from the eyes of humans and free to dream of having been born a girl.

Moreover, the island I grew up on criminalized queerness, and it was common to turn on the radio or open the paper and find pundits decrying the horrors of homosexuality. Although I didn't fully understand my queerness growing up—I didn't even know the word *transgender* until college in Florida—I knew I felt like I was a girl and that I liked boys and girls alike. But I was afraid that if I had too much attention on me, too much fire drawing the eyes of others, I would be seen as a biblical abomination, facing fists, rocks, or a different kind of conflagration altogether: hellfire appearing beneath my feet, ready to incinerate me for my sins. If fire, in my loose thinking then, represented courage, I didn't feel anywhere close to being a fire-girl.

And yet I was so drawn to that glimpse of lava flow.

Perhaps there was logic to this elemental magnetism, both then and on the road now in Hawaii. The Caribbean's volcanoes had likewise created their islands in fits of creative fury. While I didn't grow up with a volcano deity myth from our own Indigenous peoples, the Arawaks and Caribs, the volcanoes' power was obvious, from the dark rock to its black-sand beaches, and some were still active. I feared lava, understandably, yet yearned, as the watcher yearns for new planets to swim into their ken, to see its apocalyptic glow, the destroyer-of-worlds grin of whatever deity our volcanoes held.

But I was also no longer the person I'd been back then, no longer the same person I'd been even just a year earlier. As a child in that helicopter, I'd been a girl no one yet called a girl, for I was a trans girl who didn't even yet know the word *transgender*; now, two decades later, I was living openly as a queer woman married to another woman, my mountain home in Dominica replaced with an apartment in Queens after my mother rejected my coming out and told me not to return home.

And the metamorphoses went beyond transitioning. I was shifting in more elemental ways. I was slowly being reshaped, as fire alters all it touches, as lava goddesses remake their lands. I was beginning to realize that my ideas of who I was had been too small.

I'd realized this after a series of psychedelic journeys, which began a year before our trek to the volcano. At the time, I'd never taken psychedelics before, and my wife and I ended up trying psilocybin mushrooms on a whim one day, thinking it would just be a fun, weird afternoon. From that first trip, though, my life changed. Once a girl who had been nervous about surrendering control to anything, least of all a mind-altering substance—lest I do something dumb and end up being hurt or humiliated—I now found myself in love with entheogens and began to learn how to let go of those control-freak tendencies. For the first time, I felt not alone and individual in a pitiless universe, but at one with it. And I felt a sense of profound, childlike wonder at everything.

But on that first trip, I'd also had a vision, unexpectedly, of a woman, a figure draped in slithering creatures like some Minoan snake goddess, whose eyes glowed like fire, whose entire presence, as it were, felt like an energetic flame. She was creativity personified, yet she also felt casually capable of destruction, able to do anything she needed at any moment. She seemed like some self-aspect I'd never met, a version of me who was bold, unafraid, high-energy, grinning with the wild abandon of an anime character, full of awe at things everyday and extraordinary alike. After this, I sensed there was a new part of me I was capable of embodying—but it also felt so difficult.

For most of my life, you see, I've been soft-spoken, anxious, prone to living under the blue jazz of melancholy. I never imagined I could be like that incandescent snake goddess. So I began trying to integrate this new part of me, which, in turn, meant confronting the fears that had held me back for so long.

And yet, as we drive to that volcano, that forge out of which life and death alike bloom-burst, I feel like something powerful is approaching, connected, in some way, to that psychedelic vision.

I feel like a water woman learning, slowly, to fall in love with fire.

But I also feel nervous, both about what sights might await us and about the very fact that I am changing. I wonder, you see, if a person can change so much that they cease to be recognizable.

//

I remember what happened when I tried to stand out.

I remember kids snickering at my mumbling stutter when I tried to read aloud in secondary school and thinking I loved reading but was terrified of reading aloud. I remember being called "retarded" because I was awkward and spoke quietly. I remember being at my cousins' house one day playing N64 and a kid getting angry at my incompetence and calling me mentally retarded, then taking it back, saying that wasn't cool. The implications of that haunted and hurt me for years, wondering if everyone saw me like that, wondering if it would be any different if I'd been born a girl, or if I should just wish I hadn't been born at all.

I remember an older kid watching me one day in school and asking loudly with a grin if I was really a girl. And the stupid thing was how much I wanted to hug him, but instead I cursed him and shoved him and prepared to have the shit kicked out of me, but then a teacher walked by and the kid just laughed and left.

I remember my mother telling me that men couldn't grow long hair without it looking pretty, so I shouldn't try, remember her telling me if I *did* grow it I could never wear it down around others, lest they think me that worst of things, a girl. I remember telling my parents on the phone that I thought I was a girl and that it was the hardest thing in the world to tell them and that I couldn't keep it in anymore. I remember their incredulity, their telling me not to transition. I remember my father telling me on my couch that I looked like a man and would never pass. I remember my mother crying, over and over, knees up, face pressed into her legs, asking why I have done this to her, what is wrong with me, don't I know how much people will laugh at her back home with a crazy son like me.

I remember when I decided to try dating as a trans woman and a man on OkCupid sent me a message, calling me a goddess, a woman whose beauty he said he wanted to worship; it was baroque, but I felt flattered, and I told him I was trans just to make sure he knew. He never replied. An hour later, he'd blocked me. I remember telling other men who expressed interest online that I was trans, something my profile said explicitly, and the way they likewise went silent, then blocked me, perhaps with a final "Fuck you, faggot" before leaving.

I have so rarely felt confident, I realize, as I write this. To gain any confidence—would anyone recognize me then?

//

Pelehonuamea, the Indigenous people of the Hawaiian Islands called her, or *ka wahine ʻai hōnua*, the woman who devours (Pele for short, at least to her familiars). It was an apt epithet for a goddess of fire, whose hunger, like flame itself, has no bounds. This sublime power is partly why she appears prominently in the *moʻolelo*, or the foundational, still-told stories and mythos of Hawaii.

In many versions of her story, Pele is born not in the Hawaiian archipelago, but on Tahiti as the daughter of deities. Each of her siblings is associated with some natural force, like the ocean or clouds. Pele is immediately attracted to fire, an elemental bond encouraged by one of her uncles, who teaches her to control her prodigious powers. In little time, Pele is an adept at fire. In one story, Pele's proficiency angers her sister, the sea goddess Namakaokahaʻi, who jealously chases Pele from Tahiti to the Hawaiian Islands, continually dashing water on her flames; in another, Pele prompts her sister's fury by having an affair with Namakaokahaʻi's partner.

Either way, Pele arrives in Hawaii, but her sister is still incensed and eventually kills her—or so Namakaokahaʻi thinks. Pele, however, is so strong that her spirit survives the water-assault and decides to settle in Kīlauea, where her volcanic eruptions help to shape the islands as we know them today.

At some point, in many myths, she meets Kamapuaʻa, a charismatic but easily angered shape-shifting god associated with hogs, water, and certain plants. Kamapuaʻa, enamored by Pele's celestial beauty, tries to woo her, but she rejects his advances. They have a titanic battle, Pele shaking and burning the earth, Kamapuaʻa shifting forms to redirect her lava and using water to counter her blaze. Neither can defeat the other. Exhausted yet exhilarated, they briefly become lovers.

Soon, though, Pele leaves him, realizing that she wants to be alone with her beloved fire. Their breakup involves a literal breaking up: splitting the Big Island, with Pele ruling one side, her fires keeping it drier, while Kamapua'a takes the other, filling it with rainfall and greenery. This myth elegantly explains Hawaii's environmental diversity, and Pele gets to be with her first love, fire. She does not compromise; she simply embraces her nature.

Pele's biography is also, in a sense, a biography of fire itself. While fire—and lava—consumes whatever it can and is often defined as a destructive force, it does not really destroy; instead, it reshapes, restarts, transmutes wood into ash, stone into liquid, homes into memories. Certainly, such acts can feel awful, the ease with which it devours terrible. But, like the Death card in tarot, fire is ultimately a changer rather than an eliminator. In this reading, fire is more akin to an alchemist, a sorceress violently reweaving the world. The ash and smoke are still the wood in a deeper sense, just remolded into a new form—just as nothing in the universe is truly created or destroyed, just reshaped. To not live is to be frozen, unchanging; fire, by representing mutability, represents life, at least from a safe distance.

Like Pele, fire is also a wanderer, an impulse to be any- and everywhere, in the way a flame at one end of a stick slinks like an orange-blue caterpillar down to the other, or a circle of gasoline lit in one place near-instantly becomes lit throughout. Yet there are environments fire wishes to be, places it blooms best in and where, if offered the right items, it will burn brighter; Pele, likewise, is said to bless those who offer her gifts, like her favorite flower, the ohia lehua, and, in turn, to curse those who take pieces of volcanic rock—pieces of her fire, hardened into memory—beyond Hawaii, as tourists might do with a souvenir, hexes and misfortune befalling them until they return the rocks to the islands. (Fittingly, some islanders in the diaspora have mailed pieces of the black stone back to Hawaii if things start going wrong around them.)

Pele, then, is myth made matter, and matter made myth.

When I first learned about Pele, I smiled. She struck a chord with me. She was a woman of such unabashed power, a woman unafraid to blaze brightest in the dark, a woman unafraid to stand out. And she defied certain silly gender stereotypes, namely the old notion, especially common in the West, that certain elements are more appropriate for certain genders and that fire is "more" masculine. This cultural stereotype didn't apply to Pele at the time of her mythic creation, yet for me, who grew up with such gendered assumptions and a fear of being noticed, Pele seemed to trans gender, to burn the fences of conservative stereotypy. And, in an age of polarization when we are so often expected to hold one clear opinion on every topic, Pele was a far more human embodiment of opposites, a mythopoetic *coincidentia oppositorum*, whose furious devastation of the land led, in turn, to new, peaceful beginnings.

She was, in short, a vision of the kind of unconstrained woman I wished to be.

She would later, in her own ways, remind me of the Buddhist goddess Chinnamunda—whose Hindu counterpart is the very similar Chinnamasta—a figure often depicted, somewhat alarmingly, with her own severed head in her hands, blood streaming into her mouth, vampire-like, from people around her, while the blood from her neck likewise streams into everyone else's mouths. The image is symbolic: She takes life, betokened by blood, but also gives her own lifeblood to others.

Pele, like those Asian goddesses, can represent both light and dark, and that most mystic-and-language-defying of things, light-in-dark. They take; they also give. They curse; they bless. They are our proverbial dark sides, our shadows, so to speak, and also our highest aspirations. They represent a radical freedom to be—and I loved that.

I knew I wanted to feel more comfortable with all sides of me. I wanted to walk in boldness, as Byron's woman walks in beauty. I wanted to feel equally free to share my best moments, like the day of my wedding, and my worst, like the delirious afternoon I stood on the far edge of a C train station in Brooklyn, intending to jump when the train roared by, so convinced I was unlovable and that my body would always be rejected that I almost killed myself.

I wanted to talk, without shame, about all of me.

But to talk openly about mental health as a trans person is risky. Reveal that you are trans, and someone will inevitably say you are suffering from a delusion, a derangement, a disorder that makes you dangerous to yourself and others. Talk openly about your mental health, like my depression, and people nod their heads, unsurprised, for even those who support us instinctively associate being trans with mental health struggles. The more you reveal, the likelier you will be tarred, publicly or privately, as a crazy person, a person people are kind to out of the pitying deference certain able-bodied people show the disabled. To reveal that I'd been suicidally depressed in the past, or that I'd been called "retard" for years, or that I'd had a life-changing psychedelic vision—I felt scared sharing all of these out of the fear that people would stop taking me seriously, would write me off as someone with problems. And this is partly because our lives are still portrayed too simply, too linearly, in the mainstream media.

So often, when the media does offer us space, the focus is on our gender journeys, our social and physical transitions. The story begins with our realization of being queer; after we transition, the story ends, the rest of our lives supposedly a happy ending, minus the discriminations our diligent audiences know we will face, or, rare though it is, a detransition. While this focus on gender-journeying is understandable, it ultimately reduces us to those gender journeys. It elides who we are in any more complex sense. This is all the starker if our transitions are not neat moves from Gender Point A—say, "male"—to Point B—say, "female"—but less linear, less clear, sometimes contradictory transformations, less transition than transfiguration.

If we spoke of transitioning less as a move from distinct points than as a lifelong journey, a series of unpredictable peaks like an island's backbone, then it would be truer—yet to speak in this way is to contradict the rigid categorizing, cleaving impulses of America and the West more broadly, whereby everything must be individually defined and delineated.

What is water cannot be fire. Categories are not to be crossed, unless you make new subcategories. I used to live by this impulse to categorize. One of those transformations I mentioned? No longer buying into that, but trying to embrace a worldview at once more fluid and fiery, something more able to contain my own contradictions, my oddities.

I am beginning to understand fire differently, and, in turn, myself differently, not because I am shifting from one element to another—as if anyone could be just one!—but because I am expanding my view of what I contain, of what I can be.

I am beginning to acknowledge my own fire, my flames that dance like water.

//

By the time of our night drive, we've already been in Hawai'i Volcanoes National Park for a few hours. Although we're staying in an Airbnb about two hours from the volcano, and we'd loosely imagined our first full day being a gentle introduction to the island's rhythms, we worry that we might miss our chance to see lava if we wait. So around noon, we speed toward Pele's home.

As soon as we get to the visitor center—a building facing the mountain and its enormous caldera, with a huge glass wall facing Kīlauea—we see a little cascade of lava in the distance. Having forgotten our binoculars, I'd purchased the only available pair still in the shop—pink plastic binoculars for children. I trade them with my wife as we walk a maundering trail down the mountain, hoping to get as close to the lava as we can. The gastric stench of sulfur fills our noses. As we descend, we begin to hear the lava as well, for it emits a distinctive, if subtle, mix of gurgling, hissing, and crackling. Though the sky was bright when we began our trek, mist soon began to curl behind us, like some phantasmal stalker. By the time we decide to hike back up to our car, it's drizzling, gray clouds obscuring the volcano for anyone who arrives after us. When we get back up to the visitor center, a throng of tourists has filled the building, complaining about the clouds having thwarted their own chances to see the lava. Had we delayed our trip by just a little, we'd have missed that wondrous little lavafall.

Our dream, though, had been to see the spectacular show of lava burning in the dark.

We drive for a few more minutes toward where we think the lot for the volcano viewing is, the traffic slowly increasing, and then, as we round a corner, everything suddenly changes. My wife yells and points at the sky.

The clouds, once gray, have suddenly become an ominous, chthonic red, as if they are the backdrop to some apocalyptic painting, or the sky above Dante's entrance to hell. It's as if we have stepped through a doorway into another world, some eerie, eldritch place where dreamthings are forged. I feel, suddenly, in the presence of something ancient, something sublime both in its splendor and terror. We still can't see the volcano itself or its lava just yet over the endless line of rainforest trees, but the volcano's presence—*her* presence—has already become undeniable.

The parking lot, it quickly becomes clear, is full. The park rangers, who are directing people into the small lot, tell us to turn around and try again later. But the line of traffic behind us is long, and there's nowhere else to park, so as we begin to drive off, I tell my wife we should just park on the side of the road and walk back down. When we turn off the car, it's pitch-black, and we make it back down to the volcano with a flashlight.

Despite our illumination, the park rangers are furious that we walked down the dark road, lest we had stumbled, somehow, into the distant lava. "When most people fall into the volcano," one says, "we don't send a rescue team anymore. We send a recovery team for their bodies." After this unexpectedly funereal image,

I tell them the truth—that we just desperately want to see this once-in-a-lifetime display—and they begrudgingly let us in.

When we make it past the swarm of cars and tourists lining the cliffside, we finally see it. The caldera, a dark expanse of stone in the daytime, has transformed; now, tendrils of lava snake their way through the rock, steam rising slow from the orange, hovering like new ghosts. At the furthest end of the caldera, a cascade of lava viscously tumbles, like water in slow motion. The sky above the caldera is alternately red and orange, smoky-dark like a night of a thousand fireworks. The lava gleams in the black.

I stare, bewitched, for it is witchery, indeed. I am not looking at lava, not looking for some brief Instagram opportunity, not checking off a list. I am at the temple of something old. I am before a goddess—and I feel it in the thrill coursing through me, the feeling that for all its beauty, for all the safety mechanisms humans have made through barricades and park rangers and crowd-capping parking lots, we are still just as vulnerable before her wrath. That we stand here now grinning and taking pictures is because she has allowed us to; we could all so easily be wiped out, our bodies becoming part of some new land once the lava cools. How unthreatening and mundane these safety mechanisms, these orderly expeditions, can make such things feel.

I feel as though I understand something as I revel in her awful beauty. She, like me, is a monstress, a being as much angel as devil. She is queer in the way that queerness burns through the margins of things. She is Death, out of whose robes new things bloom. She is a starforge. She is Blake's Tyger, burning bright in the night. She is Borges's Aleph, a point in space in which you can see all other points in space. She is bold, radical freedom. She is, I think, someone I am coming to understand—but whom I could not have fully understood until that moment in life.

Someone's elbow jostles mine. The dream drops. I see the tourists taking photos and laughing again. We turn around to head back under the clouds' Lovecraftian hue, past a kid with hands in his pockets loudly complaining that the lava isn't cool. The park rangers glower as we walk by them with our flashlights back onto the lightless road.

I turn back one more time before getting into the car, gazing at the clouds. I still feel small, vulnerable, mortal before a myth who still lives. A goddess in a temple of mountain. A goddess for an age that has forgotten goddesses, yet whose wrath we still fear in the memory of our bones.

I thank Pele quietly for letting us see the merest hint of her power and for letting us leave in peace. I know, as I get into the vehicle, I won't forget this lava, either.

//

Halfway into the trip, I get a text from my half sister that my father has COVID and is in the hospital in Dominica. An invalid with diabetes and difficulty walking, my father is in danger anytime he gets sick. My mother, who is the source of the info my sister has, still hasn't texted me.

I message my mother frantically, mentioning in passing where my wife and I are. She only responds, as usual, by asking about money and jobs. "Hawaii," she says. "Why are you there? For work?" She never says a word about my dad. Only through my half sister can I get updates. My mother, refusing to recognize that I am her daughter, refuses to share things with me beyond recriminations, criticisms about how much money I make, or pleas to come back to Jesus.

In my anger, I buy a joint in a small, dimly lit shop. As the smoke unfurls, I peer at the landscape of trees so like the ones I grew up with. I was scared of mind-altering drugs when younger, when my mum called me by a male name and I answered. Now I cherish what plants like cannabis can offer, what they can teach us. Now I am blowing smoke, name changed, legal gender changed, the elements of my life changed. I truly would be unrecognizable to my mother, I realize, were she to see me now.

Calmer, I text her again gently for updates on my dad, but she doesn't reply. I tell her she doesn't deserve to keep this from me. No reply.

The next day, I feel furious. I want to shake the earth like Pele, make the dirt bubble in heat. At some point, we realize we'd left a pair of diving boots on a snorkel boat, so I drive to the tour company's office; in my blind rage, I almost run into a pickup at a stoplight.

Eventually, I learn from my sister that my dad has recovered. I'm grateful, but also, I finally know, beyond a doubt, that I've lost my parents. I still write to them, sometimes, but it is like writing to strangers. I'm not happy with it. It hurts. I hate the fact that I have to even wonder if my mother would tell me if my dad died.

But I accept it, and let the pain pass through me, redirecting it into energy. This, I've learned, is what fire is; it is allowing any- and everything to become kindling, a source of light. In this way, fire is a form of healing, forcing you to acknowledge, confront, and accept your Jungian shadow—your fears, suppressed feelings, pain—and, in turn, transforming them into fuel for your growth.

To be whole is to integrate your shadow—that is, to accept all of you. To destroy the future you fear and create, in the fire of *now*, the foundation of a new one, as Pele created the islands' future shapes.

This doesn't stop the pain, completely. But I am readier to live with it, and to find light in its lightlessness. I am ready to be proud of my weirdness, my queerness so strong that I was driven from one world to another, perhaps not unlike a certain goddess. I am readier to destroy the timid churchboy my past thought I would become; a wild, grinning woman stands in his place, eyes lit like the stars in the night's hair, free to self-determine, lifemaps marvelously open.

//

Later on our trip, we hike through a scrubland desert. Centuries earlier, Pele's rage flowed through here, her Rapunzelian tresses of fire stretching across the land; now, those volcanic tresses have cooled, darkened, tightened into rock we walk over. Over hundreds of years, the lava trails have taken on the textured look of old tree bark or pachydermatous skin; in some areas the lava seems to swirl, like little whirlpools frozen in time. Yet the impression I have first is of great lengths of hair.

Hair is fitting, for throughout this walk you can find thin locks of gold, remnants of volcanic activity charmingly called Pele's hair. And they look like strands of hair indeed, strewn haphazardly along the hike in rock crevices, or against hillsides, or simply along the sand. My mother, I think later, berated my long hair; Pele, gloriously, strewed her tresses across the islands.

While this desert is famous partly for being an unusual environment in the tropical isle and for Pele's hair, it is most famous for the signs you can find of Hawaiians fleeing the lava, a few of whom left footprints in the ground once the magma had cooled enough to walk on. The footprints are discussed on a sign and shown in a replica in a structure midway through the walk, but the actual footprints along the hike are hidden, so as to prevent vandals from cutting them out of the stone. You can find them only if you search.

As I walk with my wife along the lonely, quiet path, the dry brush stuporous in the sun, I feel a sudden sense of presence again, as I did before the glowing caldera. I begin to feel, in the sandy isolation, that the past is still present, that those who made those elusive footprints still linger in some way, phantasmal memories. It is a feeling at once reverential and scary. Once again, I feel small. A current of anxiety prickles down my spine.

In the past, anxiety was a constant companion. I gave in to it easily, spiraling into anxiety attacks. Now, instead, I channel my anxiety into something positive. "A demon means anything which hinders liberation," Machig Labdrön, the founder of Chöd Buddhism, famously claimed. My work with my shadow is work with my demons—not to exorcise them, for they are aspects of me, but to learn from them, instead, how to be free from an unnecessary attachment to them.

I ask myself what I'm afraid of. I imagine encountering it, imagine letting the experience pass through me. I then picture my heart as a flame, fed by the anxiety into energy, into courage, into power.

This is one of the new techniques I'm working on as I try to learn from my shadow, my fears of being hurt, of being lonely, of being overwhelmed by *what-ifs*, of standing out. And by listening to what my shadow is trying to tell me—because it always is helping me, in its own way, see how to become my best, strongest self—I'm becoming a version of myself I feel better about, both by learning how to process my emotions anew and by being open to experiences I once would've dismissed, like these mystical moments with Pele and these ghosts.

Pele is not a deity I grew up with, yet there are so many connections—terrain, vibes, broad histories of colonialism—that I feel almost at home in Hawaii, and I feel a visceral connection to the power of a volcano spirit. It does not matter, in a way. What matters is remembering that myths still walk the world with us, irrespective of culture or borders, still as powerful, despite the fortress of our beliefs, as they once were. Odysseus still sails when you drift far enough; the siren song that forced him to tie himself to a mast, ears stuffed up, still echoes on certain nights when the lanterns flicker without wind. When a twig cracks in a forest we thought we were alone in, the Old Ones still rise from memory. Pele still holds our lives in her hands. We do not need to believe in any religion—I do not—to feel the wild presence of a fire deity, the presence of one who dances with skulls beneath her feet. We *are* language, *are* story, always able to be revised, reformed.

And, in a cosmos where all, truly, is one, we can all, at some point, be another, be dust, be Death, or be an old fire goddess in the night.

DESIRE

ON BEAUTY

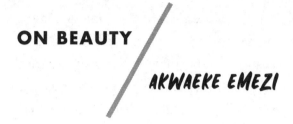

AKWAEKE EMEZI

Beauty was something that was given,
and it could just as easily be taken away.

It was so much easier to hold beauty once I stopped existing.

Before then, I had spent exhausting years trying to cope with my own embodiment, trying to untangle my gaze from that of everyone else around me. My view of my beauty was rarely mine; it was fed to me by other people, and I believed them because they were the ones looking at me. I existed in their eyes. If my family mocked me for being fat as a child, then that was true. If the cool girls in secondary school ranked me as pretty, then that too must have been true. Beauty was something that was given, and it could just as easily be taken away.

When I was sixteen, I came to the US for college, crashing into a new and hungry gaze, and I learned fast. Beauty was whittling myself down with anorexia and the gasps of college friends at the beauty of my bones through my skin. Beauty was hair whispering past my shoulder blades, straight or not, as long as there were inches and inches of it. Beauty was a formula favored by genetics—clear skin caught in the golden hour, a symmetrical face, even teeth gleaming in a smile. Like everyone else raised as a girl, I was conditioned to believe that some beauties of the flesh were more vital than others. You could be forgiven certain things if you held on to others. You could walk away from one beauty, like an unblemished body, and straight into another beauty, tattoos wrapped around limbs, metal piercing through cartilage. A palace of beauty with many rooms, and I became dizzy as the years passed and I kept falling through doorways. I still wander through a bramble of beauties, resisting some and conforming to others.

After I had top surgery, there was no way for beauty to latch itself to my body without another truth attached—that I was deviant and everyone would be able to tell when they looked at me. The bramble thickened, and old voices whispered that thinness would temper it, something that can be controlled, beauty that can be forced. It's all a delicate balance, especially as a public person, tens of thousands of eyes on you. Some beauties give you power in some palace rooms. Some beauties will make people be kinder to you, less violent. Which choices do you make? Which doorways do you throw your body into? At the end of the day, the standards are rooted in white supremacy, and the world will applaud your bones.

When I ask myself what beauty is in my eyes, the answer is that I would prefer not to have eyes. I would prefer not to have flesh, I would prefer to be dust, free of the whole thing altogether. I become ensnared by other rooms in the palace, rooms that have nothing to do with me. Yellow strokes of plaster over a wall, speck-led green vines, a sun splitting into pieces between twenty feet of waving bamboo. The sky is a riot of pink and blue and clouds, mir-rored on a lake so the horizon is consumed. The beauty is my life, that I can see these things. The beauty is that it will all end, and *that* is the most terrible beauty of all.

What could be more beautiful than the sheer vastness of noth-ing? I would throw away my existence in the effort to experience it, this magnificent promise. I have tried to throw away my exis-tence for it, and even the ritual of that was beautiful, beyond flesh, beyond my gaze or anyone else's, beyond structures and a cruel society. It was lying in a swamp watching the sky as grams and grams of medication seeped into my blood, reeds and water hum-ming softly around me. I am so temporary, like everything else, and that amplifies the beauty of the void, an inverse reflection of sorts. It all means so little in comparison, a crumbling palace, beautiful because it will die. I survive my suicide in the swamp, and I am reminded that the void is—in the end—an unattainable beauty. By the time I get there, I won't exist enough to perceive it, which feels right, to only experience the beauty of nothingness by becoming part of it myself. While I live, all I can do is imagine it, dream of it as I wait for it.

I am still never fully clear on whether my gaze on my flesh belongs to me or whether it's something I ate from someone else, swallowing down their stories. The uncertainty will remain; I don't exist enough to believe in an essential self. I have beautiful masks that I built up in palace rooms, that I know are beautiful because the audience says so, and doesn't beauty belong to the eyes naming it? My years of childhood training mean I know how to borrow people's eyes. In the mirror, sometimes they belong to my mother and brother, or those of strangers, bullies and supplicants both. Sometimes the eyes are indifferent, mechanical, assessing the body as rudimentary meat. All of it is always temporary, dust holding form until it returns to dust. Beauty sifts through my fingers like crumbled skin, and I taste the edge of sublime at the end of a lifetime.

There will be nothing as beautiful as nothing.

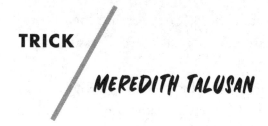

TRICK

MEREDITH TALUSAN

I didn't want you as much as what you represented.

It was with you that I discovered my womanhood. Before the night we met, I was a man who dressed up in girls' clothes. Or no, maybe I was already a woman, except I didn't know it yet. Or maybe I was halfway there, three-quarters, four-fifths, nine-tenths. How much does the rest of you need to know something before your conscious mind can perceive it?

We met during my scientist-turned-aspiring-visual-artist period on a frigid night after the century turned, when conjuring flesh out of pixels was in its infancy and one couldn't just pull connection out of air. You had to use physical wires attached to a device, which made a screeching robot sound before a voice declared, "You've got mail!," so ubiquitous that it became a Hollywood movie title.

I clicked on your message: "Ten inches and I know how to use it."

I remember the ten inches because I remember the arousal, the hardness, the thrill of catch and release. You attached no evidence because pictures weren't compulsory yet. I assumed you rounded up.

I don't remember the mechanics between the message and the ring on my intercom, just the fleeting memory of the landline, where you must have said you couldn't host, and I told you to come to my studio where I took pictures, often of men who came to my studio.

You were not attractive in the conventional sense, your features undistinguished, your body soft. But you walked into the room like you deserved the world. I found it breathtaking, the heterosexuality of it. You acted ready to save or devour a damsel in distress. I didn't want you as much as what you represented, a kind of man I couldn't catch just three months before, when I wasn't in heels and sparkly jeans, lip gloss and eyeshadow.

You tried small talk the way I'd been learning men did, so they could pretend to be interested. "Nice place." "What brought you to Boston?" "Getting cold, huh?"

"Should we cut to the chase?" I asked.

"Just the kind of girl I like." I wished you weren't so trite.

I'd set up an air mattress in a corner nook, but you had no plans to fuck horizontal. You faced me close and pointed to the floor. I knelt and you unzipped. You did not round up.

"Like what you see?" you asked in your skin-flick dialogue. *Like* was not the word I would have used, but I nodded, because I'd never had anything so big in my mouth, and the overachiever in me wanted to scale you.

It wasn't so bad in the dark, my thirst for flesh I tried to conjure through your musty odor, a pheromone mixture whose attraction I could never predict. Yours turned out below aver-age, not repulsive enough to reject but not something I would smell on my own. Nonetheless, to abort would have meant clear disappointment—for both of us—so I soldiered on.

Your taste was not unpleasant, your size I couldn't help but connect to the American dream born of my brainwashed Philippine childhood: Big Macs, Jumbo Slurpees, oversized Cadillacs. I appreciated your length and Coke-can girth in my mouth, another brand embedded in my colonized mind.

Not wanting you too much, I experienced both desire and running commentary. Blow job as American metaphor: *It's so big and featureless and pale.* Blow job as Catholic rejection: *If Sister Marietta could see me now!* Blow job as physics problem: *If the volume of a cylinder is pi times the radius squared times length, can my throat really be ten inches long?* The last became more prominent as I went on, imagining where all that volume was going as my head fell into rhythm and my throat opened up.

"Yeah, good girl, uh-huh, you like that? You like that, uh-huh, yeah, good girl?" you chanted, amid various combinations of *uh-huh*, *yeah*, *you like that?*, and *good girl*, each one repeated like hackneyed ritual. Maybe that's why I didn't feel my own resistance, not until your own jerks got violent enough that the volume had nowhere to go and my throat constricted. I reeled back.

"You can take it," you responded, while your open palm stopped my head and pushed against me when I resisted. There was a moment, a few seconds or less, when I wasn't sure, before I caught my breath and kept going. You were right, but just because I could take it, didn't mean I wanted to. I'd expected to want to, thought I'd wanted to, but there welled in me a nascent distress

I hadn't expected, a shriveling at being trapped even though I hadn't tried to escape.

That's where my womanhood was. I didn't know it then, but that was where it was.

The man in me liked this domination. The man in me who dressed as a woman had been called worse things—"filthy whore," "dirty bitch," "stupid slut"—and I enjoyed the impersonation. So when you said, "You can take it," and didn't give me a choice, and I did take it and kept taking it until I felt tears on my cheeks, drool around my lips, pain in my jaw and knees, I thought I liked it. Or maybe I did like it. A third of me liked it, a quarter, a tenth; how little can you like something and still like it?

That's the question I face now, and in the intervening twenty years. How much of a man was I then that I still liked being cornered into sexual acts, my boundaries tested, me enjoying the challenge? Because in the days, weeks, years that followed, among the few dozen men who'd been inside my mouth in those first few months of dressing, the moment when I gagged on you and you kept me from backing up is the moment that remains inside me like a hook or anchor. It has taken this long to figure out why, but now I know that when I trace my shift from man to woman, that moment was when I first noticed the momentous weight of my new gender.

The man in me didn't mind the restraint, but the woman in me seized.

//

For you see, the man in and outside of me was just living his life, happily partnered with another man for going on five years, a loving and open relationship. I was oblivious to the notion that a woman lurked somewhere inside me, schooled as I was in the logic that two entities could not occupy the same space. I used this logic while working in a cognitive science lab at MIT, figuring out how to teach computers to see like humans while nurturing my artistic ambitions at night, keeping a studio several MBTA stops away.

A cosmetics company gave the lab close to a million dollars to study how humans perceive makeup. This became my job, to understand how and in what conditions humans found women desirable when they wore cosmetics. This involved dozens of hours studying the literature on feminine attractiveness, papers like "Perceptual Asymmetries in Face Judgments" and "Vertical and Horizontal Proportions of the Face in Young Adult North American Caucasians." I also used my budget to order thousands of dollars of makeup and photo equipment to study and document the effects of cosmetics on skin. In analyzing how these effects worked in practice, it only made sense to experiment on myself.

I already knew I was mistaken for an attractive woman whenever I wore makeup; I'd known this every Halloween since college. But I had been too busy and guileless to absorb this reality's full implications, not until my MIT-funded research led me to the logical conclusion that if I was hopelessly attracted to straight men and that such men perceived me as a straight woman with just gloss, eye shadow, and a dress, then I could use makeup to lure such men into sex.

Not much luring to be done, it turned out. It only took a one-line ad and a picture. My fetish for masculine heterosexuality had a complement in straight men—the fetish for "she-males," "chicks with dicks," and "ladyboys." And as I began to meet up with men like you—doctors and plumbers, sergeants and construction workers—it was hard to know who was the fisher and who was the fish. While I reveled in catching straight men who would have ignored, taunted, or bullied me as a boy, they feasted on their fantasy of a creature, because they did treat me like a creature, who made a convincing woman until she took her clothes off, who was ready to do all the dirty things they only dreamed about, using the tools of her trade.

This convenient arrangement, this mutual fetish between man and man, lasted several months through hookup after hookup, trick after trick. It lasted until you forced me to gag.

//

That gag made me breathless.

Being breathless made me vulnerable.

Being vulnerable turned the moment dangerous.

The danger made me reel.

Your hand against my head concerned me.

That you kept it there scared me.

That you pushed after my resistance terrified me.

Your push made me want to stop.

Your push made me want to scream.

Your push made me want to run.

Your push made me want to die.

But only for a moment, because I liked being told what to do. I liked dirty things being said to me. I enjoyed the danger of sex, its unpredictability. I enjoyed my boundaries being tested, even if I didn't know them ahead of time.

But that I was not my only I. A second i lived in me, and that i was also me, except a woman.

If the first I told myself "This is exciting," while the second said, "This is dangerous," then one must be the man who decided to dress up in girls' clothes to lure straight men into bed and didn't mind a little force, while the other must be the woman who under no circumstances could allow someone else to control her body against her will.

There were more encounters after that, over the course of months, then years. Except that over time, the woman i began to take over. The woman i took greater care in picking whom to put in her mouth. She looked out for warning signs; she was more cautious, even when caution never guaranteed that she wouldn't get the kind of man who enjoyed luring women, even when I was once a man who enjoyed luring men but never, under any circumstance, would have forced a man to gag against his will.

A little of that man remains. I feel him when he tells me not to use words that sound anything like what rhymes with *ape* or *nape* or *tape*, or to use a word that sounds like *nicked him, ticked him, kicked him*—anything to avoid the letter *v*. He tells me who I was, who I am, someone who is not weak the way a woman is, not all women, but a woman who can't take just a little danger, just a little thrill, just a little unexpected force.

The little of me that's still a man keeps me calm, most of the time. But sometimes, when I'm in bed after midnight, my body seizes the way it did when I felt the force of your hand, and I remember who I am.

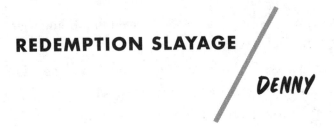

REDEMPTION SLAYAGE

DENNY

The mere possibility of hearing the applause
of an audience sometimes feels so real that
I forget what it's like to be nameless.

When I got a callback for the leading lady role in a musical re-vival Billy Porter was set to direct in New York, I sang for Porter himself.

It was the second project of his I had gotten a callback for that year, having come in for the lead of a trans rom-com for his directorial debut just months before. Despite not booking that movie, getting a second callback with him unlocked an innate feeling that maybe this would be it. He could make my life better, brighter.

After my song was over, he said, "You have a beautiful voice."

"Then give me the job," I wanted to say, though all I did was half-bow and smile bashfully.

In the elevator on my way out, I imagined what booking that

job would feel like. The mere possibility of hearing the applause of an audience sometimes feels so real that I forget what it's like to be nameless, moving through auditions and callbacks as just another person on a director's roster of actors chasing the social value that comes with being performative.

I imagine that to be praised under the bright lights would pull me from the darkness of being ordinary, let alone the darkness of being a statistic. A dead girl pronounced dead for being a girl. Or a girl not fully living because she hadn't gotten her big break.

The first singing competition my parents signed me up for was in third grade, in East Kalimantan, Indonesia. Before I went on, a producer of the event handed me a bouquet and told me to give it to one of the judges during my song. Although the added theatrics of my performance were meant to leverage my chances of winning, I placed second to a girl who stood still when she sang, and I ruminated on what my placement would have been had I let my talent speak for itself.

I had just progressed from taking over karaoke nights at my family's go-to seaport restaurant when we lived in Bali; I went from being too timid to get on the mic at the beginning of the nights to being greedy with it by the end, wanting encores for the encore itself. Prior to that, back in Jakarta, after big dinners with our extended family, I sang atop our grandparents' big leather chair, my cousins squeezed into a cuddle puddle by my feet. Whether or not my family enjoyed my one-person show, their steady gaze—albeit mostly humorous as they watched a seven-year-old belt Tamia's "Officially Missing You"—prepared me for what would be a never-ending craving to be witnessed, to feel cherished.

We left Indonesia, immigrated to the US, then moved out of Queens and settled upstate in New York. Being the flamboyant new kid, I wasn't adored by my peers the way I was by my cousins. But in eighth grade, when I sang Eric Clapton's "Tears in Heaven" for our talent show—and won—I felt a newfound respect from my classmates. I learned then how people's treatment of me shifted when I proved myself to have social value, be it my talent or accolades.

I got into the advanced choir as a freshman in high school, won a solo award for our show choir competition, and was cast in the musical plays every year. At fourteen, I discovered *RuPaul's Drag Race*, where I watched Raja Gemini, an Indonesian drag queen, win her season. I stole makeup from the theater department and learned how to apply it by watching drag queens on YouTube. Eventually, I wore makeup, skirts, and platform loafers to trigonometry class at 7 a.m., and what used to be a source of my peers' interrogation of me as the femme kid in middle school became my source of social power as a trans person by the time I graduated. Having a sense of solidity and certainty in who I was, even if half-assed and performative, protected me from harassment.

I went to college in a small upstate town called Oneonta, the kind of predominantly white public university that was politically blue in the middle of its majority-red town. With fewer than seven thousand students attending the school, being the sole openly trans girl, let alone a brown girl, separated me from an already small student body.

Clouded by the thrill of being seen, I took a fellow student's wagging finger and "Yasss" as she passed me by one morning as a compliment. I took strangers' wide smiles and nods at me as a kind gesture or an ode to my "bravery" rather than self-congratulatory tolerance of my presence. I took being on the school's magazine cover as a celebration of diversity, and not flimsy damage control atoning for the scrutiny I endured when using women's restrooms—among other challenges I faced due to my visibility. For most of my college years, I moved through campus with more people knowing me than I did them.

Despite my desire to perform in front of an audience, what I initially found flattering—being well-known in school—grew into the weight of being, or at least feeling like, an institution's mascot. I often felt like I did on that stage in East Kalimantan, adorned in flowers that weren't for me but for offering, as if showing up empty-handed dismissed me of any credibility—as if showing up as I was didn't quite cut it anymore.

//

Yazmin Vash Payne, Ty Underwood, Taja DeJesus, Lamia Beard, Shade Schuler, Ashton O'Hara, and K. C. Haggard were among the trans women of color murdered in the US during my years in college. While guest-hosting an MSNBC segment, writer-producer-director Janet Mock named these women in an effort to bring the severity of the deaths of these Black and brown trans women into the light.

"Today we learn their stories and say their names, not out of obligation but out of recognition that these women had value, had purpose, and were loved," she said. "And they will be missed."

In tandem with Mock's statements, Laverne Cox, who had been on the rise since *Orange Is the New Black*, declared a "State of Emergency" for the trans community. Just the previous year, supermodel Geena Rocero came out as trans in a TED Talk because she believed living in secrecy wouldn't do the trans community of color justice. I moved through my early college years with an acute awareness of how violent the world often was toward trans women of color, although the murder victims were mostly Black and rarely Asian.

In school, singularity made me hypervisible by default, and I took on an activist role out of fear of being without purpose. If I didn't emphasize the importance of my safety in school and in the world, how was I to know my mere presence at school merited the respect and acceptance I desperately sought? If I were hurt, or worse, how was I to ensure the administration and student body did not have an excuse for forgetting or dismissing me?

The "State of Emergency" of Black and brown trans women became my talking point across several circles in school; it was the subject of my slam poetry pieces, my US history class's final paper, my independent blog, even my open mic performances. As there was an urgency to the way I politicized being a brown trans teenager in college, there was an urgency to the way I politicized glamour, too.

In order to not feel like I was a ticking statistic, and therefore pitied, I relied, yet again, on performance. Beauty allowed me to get through school with a sense of being "above" the looming tragedy of my community, even though tragedy and my fear were already the underbelly of my academic career.

At Oneonta, I modeled myself after glamorous trans women, squeezing myself into cisnormative conventions of beauty to compensate for what often felt like my grim reality: I was not cis.

My access to normal college experiences fell short in comparison to other girls' at school because I was not cis, and even more so because I was not white. My only option, I felt, was to out-pretty the girls on campus. *I'll be respected and desired,* I thought, *and maybe the illusion of being just like them will make me happy.* Besides, who else was I to turn to if not the beautiful and successful trans women I saw in the media, like Geena, Laverne, and Janet?

Between having a strategic knowledge of makeup and owning a hyperfeminine wardrobe, I was acutely aware of how performative gender was for me. Despite being an out trans girl in college, I hoped to stand out only for being beautiful. I was flattered when strangers started to buy me drinks at the bar or held doors open for me, and I progressively craved the feeling more. I wanted to keep chasing the high of the benefits hyperfemininity gifted me, but that too became exhausting; even being glamorous required me to excel.

While the work of popular and beautiful trans women emboldens me, it seems as though I have no option but to be fabulous—and notably so—in order to feel secure as a marginalized person. I don't want to be remembered by a news headline reporting that I have been killed—but can I rely on the world to keep me safe only if I am memorable and beautiful beyond belief?

Before I transitioned, I wanted to be seen simply because of my artistic contributions. Once I understood what being trans in the US meant, I wanted to be seen because of my artistic contributions in spite of what women like me continue to endure. My shortcoming was, and sometimes still is, my belief that fame and glamour can save me.

There are many trans women of color to idolize; there are also many trans women of color to mourn. I feel inspired by the former, terrified by the latter. I want to know where to exist between the zenith of applause and funeral. I am grateful for trans celebrities because they serve as a mirror for me, and I am humbled by the victims of antitrans violence because they remind me of what I have to lose.

I grieve the girls who dreamed of blooming when all the world could offer was another headline. I mourn with the girls who go to bed under stars in the names of their lost sisters.

Sometimes I wonder if getting out of bed and brushing my teeth in the morning would be easier if I had an Academy Award–size audience cheering for me. Sometimes I find the mundane tasks of my everyday life to be excruciatingly tedious and dull.

But maybe that's the gap between glamour and death for trans women of color; a little life teetering on the edge of phenomenon and the ordinary, chasing miracles in the getting-by and finding stillness in the wonders.

SPEAKING MY LANGUAGE

EDGAR GOMEZ

At a time when we are being systematically wiped out,
the *x* in *Latinx* is about more that accuracy.

It was getting dark out in Tijuana, the streetlights along Avenida Revolución flickering to life. I hurried down the busy commercial avenue along with two girlfriends from college, the three of us seeking shelter from the storm clouds circling above us. When raindrops began hitting the asphalt ahead of us, we darted into the nearest building, rushing past the sign hanging over the front door welcoming us into Rubiks Bar. We climbed a narrow flight of stairs following the sound of clinking bottles and laughter. On the second floor, neon lights cast a red glow over a group of friends sitting at a table singing along to the Los Enanitos Verdes song playing—"Ahora estoy aquí, borracho y loco!!!"— their voices a relief after the last two tourist traps we'd been to. They, like us, might have been tourists, too, but at least here we all spoke the same language.

It was late April 2018, the tail end of spring break season. Over at the bar, I peeled a sticky drink menu off the counter, a smile slowly spreading across my face as I looked over the specials: There was a drink named after Madonna; another one was called the Trans X. The vibe was kind of giving gay bar, but you can never be too sure. Rubiks—like the cubes, I realized—had a retro aesthetic that made it hard to tell if it was actually a gay bar or just '80s-themed. For every queer thing that pointed me in one direction, like the disco ball twirling in the ceiling, there was something undeniably heterosexual, like a wobbly steel table with a *Ghostbusters* poster laminated on its surface. For all I knew, Trans X was a reference to the *Transformers* movies . . . I briefly wondered if Rubiks was one of those elusive, noncommittal third spaces, a "gay-friendly" bar, then ordered my friends a round of shots.

A good amount of tequila later, the three of us were out on the dance floor, buzzed and singing along with the crowd as the DJ moved from Gloria Trevi to Los Prisioneros to Thalía. It was getting hot inside, so I slipped off the hoodie I had on and wrapped it around my waist, feeling a little self-conscious in the tight black tank top I had underneath. Right as I was about to put my hoodie back on, one of my friends pointed out a cute guy on the other end of the dance floor staring my way. I tried not to blush. He was like Rubiks in that I couldn't really tell what his deal was, dark hair slicked back cholo style, a Virgen de Guadalupe tattoo trailing up his arm. I considered going up to him, but before I could summon up the nerve, a little voice in my ear whispered: *Careful. Don't do too much.* It was the same voice that restrained me whenever I wasn't somewhere explicitly gay. I liked to think of myself as proud and unapologetic, but in reality, I was often prone to sudden bouts of paralyzing fear in public. Two years earlier, a man in my hometown, Orlando, stepped into Pulse Nightclub and pressed down on the trigger of an assault rifle, killing forty-nine queer people, my friends. Ever since, I've had trouble feeling safe in bars. The possibility that Rubiks was gay-friendly might have defused my anxiety, but I wasn't sure.

After a few more songs, I went to the bathroom, scolding myself for not talking to the guy while I waited in line. What was the worst that could have happened? I hated how dramatic I could be, always thinking in extremes. When it was finally my turn, I rushed into a cramped stall. The dark, grimy walls were plastered with posters and graffiti. I held my breath against the stench of urine, focusing on a flyer in front of me advertising a beer bucket special, then the name of a band scrawled with a Sharpie, before my eyes settled on an old-looking sticker, glossy in patches but mostly faded by now, that said: "Orgullo Latinx."

It wasn't my first time seeing the word *Latinx*. After the shooting at Pulse, it was everywhere from celebrity Instagram posts to newspaper headlines and political campaigns. All around the country, people were using *Latinx* to encompass the multitude of identities of the 49 LGBTQ+ folks who were killed in the club on Noche Latina. I'd seen the word before Pulse, too, *Latinx* as well as its chronically online predecessor *Latin@*. In high school, I was always turning to the internet when I had questions I didn't dare ask the people in my real life: "Am I gay?" and "What if I don't feel like a boy or a girl? What does that make me?" In retrospect, I can't help but laugh at these questions, though not in a mean way, more like when I look at old pictures from those days and barely recognize myself anymore. Still, I'm grateful I had the internet to turn to. Online I discovered a whole language to express what I was feeling: *nonbinary, gender-fluid, Latin@/x.* They were just words, words I hardly ever uttered aloud much less felt comfortable claiming as my own, but they kept me company during a time of my life when I was most lost. They reminded me that though I didn't have an answer for everything, at least I wasn't alone.

That night in Tijuana, staring at *Latinx* written on the wall, I couldn't help but laugh again. It was like running into an old friend in another part of the world.

When I was growing up in Florida, no one in my family used words like *gender* and *the binary*, but the idea that there were strict, specific roles for men and women was still very clear.

The men closest to me were my *tíos*. Tough, masculine, machistas to the bone. In Nicaragua, where my mom's side of the family is from, one ran a cockfighting ring—a brutal sport that involves abusing roosters and setting them loose with knives. My tíos who immigrated to the US found jobs in construction. They worked long days doing hard manual labor, demanded my *tías* have a hot meal ready for them when they got home, then spent the rest of the night drinking in front of the TV. On weekends, some would run off to the cockfights, others to be with their secret girlfriends, or who knows where—because they didn't owe anybody an explanation.

My tías were on the opposite end of the power divide. They were expected to hold down jobs of their own, keep the children dressed and the house clean and their legs shaved, all the while answering to my tíos' every beck and call. Of course there was also a lot of love in their relationships, but as a child, what I mostly picked up on was how frustrated everyone seemed. On the outside my tías maintained an air of quiet dignity, but as soon as we stepped into a church, they would immediately drop to their knees, clasp their hands together, and break down sobbing. Some of my tíos were violent with them, especially when they were drinking. At night, I'd hear the women in my family on the phone consoling each other: "Don't listen to him. He just gets crazy because of the war," one would say, meaning the war in Nicaragua many of my tíos were forced to fight in as teenagers. Or "When he's older, he'll calm down and stop all that. Watch."

The latter was something adults frequently said about me, too, albeit for different reasons. Because I was scrawny and sensitive and preferred watching *novelas* to *fútbol*, because I cried whenever my curly hair grew too long and I was forced to cut it. In private I wondered, since I liked doing "girl things," whether that meant I *was* a girl, and maybe I'd been born in the wrong body. I didn't have any issues with the body I was born with, but because those were the options presented—you are either a male or a female—I believed I had to pick one or the other.

All I really wanted was to be myself without having to check if every one of my actions aligned with my body parts first. I could see how harmful living under these limitations was: in my tíos and their unwillingness to be vulnerable, instead drowning their sorrows with alcohol, letting their anger fester and fester inside until they exploded in fits of rage; in my tías, who had to be silent and subservient in exchange for the so-called security that having a husband offered. I naively hoped others would also agree that these narrowly defined roles hurt all of us.

Whenever I could, I tried to experiment with my own unique

mixture of masculinity and femininity. I'd hole up in the bathroom at home tweezing my eyebrows into razor-sharp lines, claiming I was imitating my favorite male reggaeton stars. At school I hung a messenger bag over my shoulder like a purse. I was popular among lots of straight boys who felt like they could open up to me without judgment, maybe because they thought of me as the best of both worlds: a boy friend they could talk to like a girl. It's funny looking back at how similar our insecurities were: *Why doesn't so-and-so like me? What if I'm not good enough? Do you think I'm ugly?* Beneath the cool-guy personas they put on for the other boys on campus, they were just as scared of the future and not measuring up to the roles they'd inherited as I was. I wish we could have stayed friends, so that we could have worked together to figure out a new way to live, but as we grew older, little by little the straight boys began keeping their distance.

I guess they realized the same thing I did: that there are real, life-or-death consequences for those who follow a different path. That queerness can get you shunned by your family or arrested by the police, or lead to your job applications being thrown in the trash. These were the early 2000s, back when the military's actual, for-real policy on homosexuality was "Don't Ask, Don't Tell," as if simply not talking about us would cause us to disappear.

Because of this imposed silencing of our community, it took me a while to find us, but gradually I did—first on the internet, where I could hide under the cover of anonymity, and once I turned eighteen at Orlando gay bars partying with drag queens, trans women, butch lesbians, people who questioned the idea that we are obligated to follow some weird rules about how we're allowed to act. Many of my new friends didn't identify with the labels of "boy" or "girl." Some used they/them pronouns to declare that distinction; others were fluid and comfortable with any pronoun. Outside of my tight-knit queer family, I tried countless, clumsy ways of explaining myself. "I'm like Walter Mercado!" Or "You know that diaspora feeling of not knowing where you belong, like *no soy de aquí, ni soy de allá?* Nonbinary is like that. I'm not masculine or feminine—I'm both." But with my people, I never had to explain. We just were.

Truthfully, I don't care if others understand who I am or what *Latinx* is. There is a lot of stuff about cis people that I personally do not get: gender reveal parties, decorating bathrooms like the beach, truck nutz. But as much as I want to make jokes about how strange it is to be human, another part of me needs my community understood—for our safety, if nothing else. People are afraid of what they don't understand. When they don't know us, they are easily manipulated into harming us. In the past few years alone, books with queer characters have been censored throughout the country; trans kids have been banned from playing sports and using the bathroom; hate crimes against LGBTQ+ folks based on gender have jumped more than 30 percent. Violence against us is so everyday that it barely makes a dent in the news anymore, like the story of the man who walked into a gay bar in Brooklyn and set it on fire. This was in 2022.

Some say that the battle over the word *Latinx* is unnecessary, since there are already the gender-neutral terms *Latin* and *Hispanic*. I am glad these exist, but that doesn't change the real point of the word. *Latinx* wasn't created just to be a more accurate description of the entire community (though yes, that is one aspect of it), but to specifically draw attention to those of us who are most at risk of violence. At a time when we are being systematically wiped out, the *x* in *Latinx* is about more than accuracy. It forces people to confront that queer people are and have always been part of the larger community, and we're not going anywhere.

//

For a six-letter word that truly just means "queer people exist," there has been a lot of backlash against *Latinx*, some of it understandable, some slightly less so, like the rumor every conspiracy-loving tío is spreading about *Latinx* being a word invented by gay lizards from space who are planning to groom all the children and brainwash them into getting socialist Brazilian butt lifts or whatever. If you are that tío, sir, please stop drinking the Fabuloso—put the bottle down.

Of all the problems people have with *Latinx*, the most reasonable to me is that it's just too hard to pronounce in Spanish, though the alternative *Latine* also exists (for this reason I use *Latinx* in English, *Latine* when speaking Spanish). Since Spanish is a very gendered language (for example, spoons are girls, *la cuchara*; forks are boys, *el tenedor*), there's an argument that it would be incredibly difficult to degender every word in a sentence and still have a natural-sounding conversation. The trouble with this, however, is that I don't know a single Latinx/e person who is advocating that we degender every word. We are not bothered that forks are boys, I promise. With Spanish, we're only saying people have the option to use *Latine* when referring to a large group of *human beings*, some of whom may identify outside the binary. If you're talking about *one individual person* who uses gender-neutral pronouns, all it takes is tweaking the word referring to them with an *e*, which we already see in neutral words like *estudiante*. If this all sounds overwhelming, just call people *amorsito* or by their name, and you'll be fine.

Others have said that the whole idea of being nonbinary and using the word *Latinx* is too academic, that it's being forced on the population by scholars and activists living in their ivory towers while the average person is worried about real problems, like rent. But to me this sounds patronizing. Why is it so hard to believe the average person is intelligent enough to think about sexuality and gender? I must be missing something, because I can't tell you how many cheap plastic lawn chairs I have sat on listening to drunk relatives fighting about communism, and Ricky Martin, and why you need to pierce the baby's ears or else people will think she's a boy. Besides, regardless of where the word originated, the people I hear using *Latinx/e* the most are young, working-class queer people of color, at community centers in Puerto Rico and flea markets in Queens and drag shows across Mexico City. And it's young, working-class queer POC who experience the highest rates of homelessness,* which makes the notion that we're only thinking about gender because we don't have real problems especially cruel and insulting. There are queer people thinking about gender *and* rent, not because they have endless time, but because their genders directly impact their ability to secure housing.

But the most popular argument I've heard about *Latinx/e* by far is that "Latinos don't even use it!" Critics of the word regularly cite the 2024 Pew Research Center poll that found that

---

* The Trevor Project, *Homelessness and Housing Instability Among LGBTQ Youth*, February 3, 2022.

"75% of Latinos who have heard of the term Latinx/e say it *should not* be used to describe the Hispanic or Latino population" and that among those, 36 percent believe "it is a *bad thing* for people to use Latinx more often."[*] (Emphasis placed by Pew.) Challengers of *Latinx/e* love to drop these statistics like it's some big GOTCHA moment, but when I hear these numbers, I'm not all that surprised. It is not a devastating new discovery to me that there is rampant homophobia and transphobia in the *Latino* community. It is not a surprise that the majority of Latinos in a country rapidly moving to repeal LGBTQ+ rights do not want to associate themselves with queerness. Several of my own family members struggle to accept that I'm gay; why would they accept *Latinx/e*? What would my life look like if I only ever did what the majority of people believed was right?

I'm not saying that all Latin people are homophobic and transphobic—though out of the ten countries with the most murders of trans people, six are in Latin America[**]—and I'm also not saying that that's why those numbers are what they are. But I am saying that we need to stop pretending these things have nothing to do with it. I'm saying *Latinx/e* is still new, the same way *Latino* was once the latest buzzword, rising to prominence in the '90s as a replacement for the more commonly used *Hispanic*. So it's only natural that some are going to be skeptical and take a minute to adopt it and that it may not even

[*] Luis Noe-Bustamante, Gracie Martinez, and Mark Hugo Lopez, *Latinx Awareness Has Doubled Among U.S. Hispanics Since 2019, but Only 4% Use It*, Pew Research Center, September 12, 2024.
[**] Lucia He, "Latin America: The Most Deadly Region for Transgender Communities," *Equal Times*, November 16, 2016.

be perfect. Latinidad itself isn't perfect; it constantly fails to capture the vast array of experiences of people from over thirty countries with differences in race and class, as if a coffee farmer in Puerto Rico and a blond, blue-eyed Cuban in Miami and an undocumented Mexican woman in LA all share the same viewpoints, have the same needs, and shoulder the same fears. Language changes. It is always shifting and adapting to suit the needs of our time, and one of the most urgent needs of today is to protect queer and trans people of color, in particular Black and Indigenous queer people, who face the highest rates of violence and policing.

It's still too early to tell whether *Latinx/e* will stick around for the long haul, or whether someone will come up with something better that everybody can agree on. Whatever its fate, I suspect that if there is a new word, we're going to have to answer questions a little deeper than what's easier to pronounce in Spanish or who said it first.

Back in the bathroom at Rubiks Bar, I wasn't thinking about the evolution of language and gender. I wasn't thinking about how I could convince the next person I met that I am not an evil space lizard. I was tipsy and thinking about the cute guy at the other end of the dance floor, hoping that if I went up to him and he turned out not to be queer, he wouldn't be the type of straight dude who has a panic attack and freaks out. Seeing the word *Latinx* on a sticker didn't promise me safety, but its presence at Rubiks did feel like a small reminder from the universe that the world is changing, slowly but surely.

A few minutes later, I reunited with my friends on the dance floor, trying to act casual when I saw my Tijuana crush nursing a beer a few feet away from them. When the DJ put on a song by The Smiths, people around the bar ran over to join us on the dance floor, pushing our bodies closer and closer together. The two of us danced separately while stealing occasional glances at each other under the blinking strobe lights, his face green and blue and red.

"Hey!" he yelled over the loud music. His hair had gotten messy in the last hour, black tendrils plastered against his forehead with sweat.

"Hey!" I yelled back.

He smiled, took a step forward, and like that, we were dancing together.

I turned to my girlfriends, who were watching and giggling. One of them winked.

We were there, dancing, for a few more songs. Then he pulled me away from the dance floor.

I love it when people don't have to say much. That's the great thing about being completely understood.

BECOMING FEMME

TANAÏS

I'd wanted this femme with my whole body,
but without the next morning's regret.

On the night of my fortieth birthday, I ended up hooking up with a beautiful West Indian femme whom I barely knew. I hosted the party in the backyard of a local bar, and most everyone was someone I'd loved for years. But this femme, they'd been one of my wildcard invites, someone I'd crushed on from afar. For most of the evening, I floated about like a butterfly, drinking Palomas, giggling and posing for photos. At some point in the night, they sat next to me. I let myself be cornered.

"I want to make you come, tonight," they said, right out the gate, eyes large, black, unblinking. Their energy felt like a flaming oil spill on my wavy, drunken waters. Not quite my style of flirting—I prefer banter, touch, the unspooling of an endless conversation, until there's nothing left to do but take your clothes off and jump into bed together. But on that night, at the age of forty, I wanted to feel intensity. I don't remember how I answered them or if I did at all, because we started kissing, ravenous for each other's lips.

My husband was only a few feet away, engrossed in conversation, not remotely aware of us going at it—not that he'd care. Even in my liquored state I knew that we needed more privacy, so I grabbed their hand, and we made our way inside. We stopped for a moment to make out, right next to my sister and family friend, who commented, "That's hot." Whereas my sister, a queer femme trailblazer, had loved, married, and divorced another queer femme, for me, it had been years since I had kissed another femme, having been with a man for more than a decade.

I've missed this, I thought.

We left the bemused pair to make our way to a booth. More kissing, licking, pressing fingers against each other's cunts through clothes. Strangers sitting next to us didn't seem to mind two South Asian femmes madly making out.

Everything about them intoxicated me, a body tighter and more supple than my own, both of us brown-skinned, black-haired, bedroom-eyed. I wore a violet faux-silk gown with the waist cut out. They scratched long acrylic nails on my exposed skin. They, too, wore purple, but a jumpsuit, in a lunar shade. She, a moon, reflecting my hot, burning light. I wanted to feel our wet cunts on each other's tongue. We were both queer, diasporic femmes, a West Indian and a Bangladeshi, our people deemed outsiders to the Indian Brahmanical dominant culture, before the British, but especially after. Forever outsiders to the pervasive, perpetual Indian center of South Asian experience. West Indians migrated across the *kala pani*, the black water of the Atlantic, whereas my people had always lived on the far Eastern frontier, a river-laden, verdant land, constantly extracted and denuded of resources and human labor, by kings and colonizers. Across time and space, borders and nations, the brown-skinned, caste-oppressed femme has long been erased from history. Nations burned in their name, as they remained a specter in the patramyth, the official record of history by the victors.

That night, with the feeling of her beauty, warm and pulsing in my hands, I felt eons between us, as I have before, with South Asian lovers.

We ended up at my apartment, along with a dozen other friends. She went up to my husband, Mojo, and said, "I'm going to fuck your wife tonight," to which he replied, nonchalantly, utterly ready for the night to be over, "Sure, whatever she wants."

My lust swallowed back up inside its cocoon. Suddenly, I wanted them to leave. I wanted everyone to leave. Eventually, they did. I spent the next hour, until dawn, on the living room couch, making myself cum, thinking of them, as my husband slept in our bedroom. I'd wanted this femme with my whole body, but without the next morning's regret, or awkwardness, as soon as our highs wore off. In another era, perhaps we would've hooked up in my bedroom, let my man have the couch, and if it were another man, not the one I married, have him join us. Introducing a third to our marriage, when no one was sober, wasn't exactly the start to forty that I'd pictured. More than anything, I wanted solitude. I remained content to reanimate this ache for another femme within the distant confines of fantasy.

I felt desirous, but simultaneously unsettled, by the distance that disappeared between them and me. With masculine people, with men, the boundary of our difference has afforded me psychic space, ultimately, affording me the space to selfishly be in my art. Even during penetration, there is a separation. I recognized what arose in me. There is a danger and wildness that femmes inhabit, which I myself inhabit, a body spilling out of a dress, a voice deepened by smoke, sweetened by estrogen, a kohl-lined stare that pierces through you. Even in our intoxicated state, this thrilled me, but unmoored me. For the first time in years, I found myself erotically charged in the presence of another femme, a boundary dissolved—but rather than let myself lose myself, I retreated.

In the afterglow of that night, I felt gratitude that my queerness continues to teach me about what my heart, body, and mind desire. Rather than tuck that evening away, as if it were a mere shimmer of youth, a fleeting encounter, I remembered how femmes conjure this innate, powerful urge to worship: a goddess, a whore, the ocean, the sun, and the night.

//

On ne naît pas femme, on le devient. One is not born a woman, but rather, becomes one. I reconsider Simone de Beauvoir's iconic words. Let me slip away from the acceptable translation of the French word *femme* as woman—let the word *femme* be supplanted by queer imagination. As in: *femme,* liberated from cisgender womanhood; *femme,* unlike the word *woman,* does not bear the weight of man on its end. I'm sensitive to language, how it looks, how it sounds, how it feels on the tongue. Femme, a queer, feminine person. *Femme,* to describe a lesbian, queer, or bisexual woman in post–World War II America, is a Western locus that never imagined femmes like us. Fast forward to the future, and femme transcends biology or anatomy—*femme* is embodied. We become femme for ourselves, for each other.

As my sister and I learned to become Bengali, Muslim, American women, we learned that the most potent currency, for us, so often felt like a monstrous impossibility—to be desirable, pure, pious, a mother, a daughter, a wife, at once. *On devient femme,* we become femme, we become who we've chosen to be, not who we were raised to be. *Femme* subverts prescribed feminine ideals. *Femme* pulses with the feminine, fierce, powerful, raging, soft, adorned, audacious, fluid—the Divine.

//

I renamed myself Tanaïs, a portmanteau of the first two letters of each part of my birth name, Tanwi Nandini Islam, a syncretic name that holds the Buddhist, Hindu, and Muslim lineages of Bengal. When the name came to me, I'd just smoked a joint; the name Tanaïs appeared in my mind's eye. My three names, in a single exhale, are free of patrilineage, religion, or language. Tanwi quite literally means a slender, young woman, but Tanaïs is femme, they, them, a return to my pre-English mother tongue, Bengali, and its genderless pronouns. As I began to publish work with this new name and corrected old friends to call me by my new name, I sensed their alienation from me; they missed their old girl, Tanwi. She wasn't dead exactly, but I was mid-rebirth. I learned that not everyone will see you through this period, because they can't actually see you. And I, too, was unable to see them, the way they deserved and wished to be seen.

Each night that I sit at my writing desk, I face that nameless, cosmic void. For most of my reading life, I encountered few examples of brown-skinned, Muslim Bangladeshi femmes in the American literary imagination. Zadie Smith's *White Teeth* featured the most alive diasporic Bangladeshi characters I'd ever read—men—in the year 2001, when I was a sophomore at Vassar, just after 9/11. I loved those characters. I need those fictive people, who felt like my people, and I knew, that one day, I would write us, too.

Imagining and recording the femmes lost to the patramyths of history is work that I've devoted myself to. Patramyths are the record of history, one that has erased the histories of the marginalized to protect systems of domination. In a culture obsessed with spectacle, fame, and mass appeal, the lives and art of marginalized people too often get absorbed by the dominant culture, without compensation or credit.

Femme, they, them: a rejection of the dominant culture's version of what it means for us to be ourselves. *Femme*, a return: to an ancestral, divine, beyond-binary self.

Does asserting myself as femme strip me of all the experiences I've lived as a woman? No. I've eschewed the parlance of our times—*nonbinary, woman, bisexual*—to describe myself. Each of those terms feels imprecise, still strangely centering a binary. Cisgender women will never be safe and free—whether we're talking access to abortion or periods or reproductive health, ending rape culture or writing literature—if nonbinary and trans and queer and femme people, all marginalized genders, are not also safe and free. *What happens to them and theirs happens to us and ours, too.* Cisgender women are not the only ones writing real women's stories and lives. We don't write and read our own stories and lives. We need to write to one another, read one another, and free one another, just as we do this for ourselves.

//

Femme is a syncretic confluence, where the rivers of queer, trans, woman, girl meet, unsplit by the sharp edges of identity, which are too often contorted into deadly crosshairs, with femmes as its perpetual target. When it comes to feminist liberation, all people of marginalized genders must share the same urgency to end patriarchal violence. We live in a time of grave, ghastly genocidal warfare, perpetrated by dictators who stoke the flames of nationalism, religious fundamentalism, and ethnomyth into a conflagration of terror. Those who've never dreamed of fighting in wars, but dreamed of their children growing up, have paid with their lives. Lineages vanished from the record. Gruesome violence is an innate aspect of our human origin story. Our ancestors fought one another to death, for land, food, shelter, and we, the living, are the descendants of the ones who survived. Nothing has changed, especially the antidote to violence, in the aftermath, which remains love: free, boundless, persistent love.

In South Asia, caste evolved to protect the wealthy, the kings, the warriors, the Brahmanical patriarchy. Goddess worship be damned; whether Abrahamic or Brahmanic, religious tenets protect men's freedom and the patramyth of their superiority.

When the Buddhist teachings of Siddhartha Gautama outwardly rejected caste or any notion of hierarchy among humans, his message spread, across Asia, across empires, along the Silk Road, for centuries, until eventually, both Hindu and Muslim conquest would wrest back power.

Raised a Muslim, I've always longed for reconnection to
the ancestral, pre-Islamic feminine divine of East Bengal, the
land now known as Bangladesh. In my practice of deity yoga, I
imagine myself as a divine femme. I concentrate on the Tibetan
Buddhist deity, Green Tara, or the Hindu goddess of death, destruction, and rebirth, Kali. In these meditations, I return to that
cosmic void. Shimmers of old acid trips morph into neon pat-
terns: damask, mandala, honeycomb. Carnal pleasure once felt
tantamount to personal freedom, which is no surprise in a South
Asian Muslim household. The liberation I seek in this era of my
life transcends the body, until there's nothing but Emptiness.

As a femme in this particular body, each and every day of
my life, I'm read as a woman and treated as one. My life partner is a light-skinned North African Irish man. In the binary
world, we are husband and wife, man and woman, but in our
personal, spiritual, secret, romantic life, Mojo and I dance the
masc-femme continuum. He first introduced me to these prac-
tices, unbound to the Islam or Catholicism of his own family,
rekindling a long-dormant ancestral connection to Vajrayana
Buddhism. Our love deepens our solo human experience. Together, we support each other's individual journeys to liberation;
we keep learning each other's soft and hard edges.

We first met on a dance floor. Within a few minutes of dancing, we started kissing, and ended up at his place. I had been with
only one other blue-eyed man before, a casual college thing;
it was a physical feature I neither worshipped nor coveted. It
kind of scared me, to be honest, the iciness of blue. I'd always
pictured myself with someone brown-skinned, black-haired,
brown-eyed—in my mind. Physical continuities between my-

self and my lover were a matter of decolonizing myself. The night of my fortieth birthday, I resuscitated that dormant desire.

Femme, as mirror, as kindred, as lover.

With another South Asian, whatever phenotypic-psychic connection we share is something I'll never know with my husband. There's a sadness I've felt about this, something so deep I can't find the reason; I just feel what I feel. No lover became kin to me, as quickly, as deeply, as Mojo. Those first days of our bond laid the foundation for a love unlike any that I'd experienced. The discordance between my fantasy mate and the one I've got is immaterial—from the minute we locked eyes, we were moved. Spirit. We are each other's lovers, each other's children, each other's parents. We've chosen not to have children in this lifetime; we've chosen to end the worldly cycle of samsara, death and rebirth. We witness each other's growth in every way, shape, and form, free to love whom we wish, how we wish. But each day, we choose to love each other, to the end.

//

Reaching for spectral ancestors and divine femme deities is but another act of mythmaking to survive the harsh reality of today's world. When I sit down to write, I think about the women in my family, the Muslim, Black, Dalit, and Indigenous femmes who weave abundance into a world that rarely ever puts respect on their names, their art, labor, intellect, or contributions. I think about my grandmothers, both child brides, who lived as British, Indian, and Pakistani citizens; only my maternal grandmother, Nanu, lived to see the birth of Bangladesh and the death of her son. When Nanu died at the start of the pandemic, in Dhaka, I never got to ask her questions I'd been too shy to ask as a young person. Who did she dream of becoming before she married? I'd never have those answers, only pieces of her: kantha quilts, a photograph, an earring, its pair lost forever.

On the other side of my family, I'd never known my paternal grandmother, my Dadi, Lutfunnessa, who married at age nine, the unjust custom of the time. Dadi died in her forties, of throat cancer, when she was just a few years older than me. My whole life I've been told that I look and carry myself like her. Only six of the children she birthed most of her adult life survived. I'd only seen a single, faded photo that had eaten away the details of her face.

When my Ma visited my ancestral home, she discovered a discarded old trunk. There's a video of my cousin breaking it open. He succeeds. Everyone gasps. Its contents created something of a confrontation; these were the sole remnants of my Dadi's life. Ma grabbed what she could, shocked that these treasures— heirlooms from the 1940s—had been neglected by her in-laws. There is a photograph of my Dadi, sitting next to my grandfather, a stern-looking man much older than her. Her deep-brown face is anything but serene; I read in her fierce eyes both fury and grief. There is a letter, written from her hospital bed, suffering, angry, and anguished at being alone, abandoned. This *objet de mort* haunted my mother, who'd been a young bride the very first time that she'd visited my father's home. I imagine she wondered what her life might've been like had she gotten the chance to know her mother-in-law.

In that trunk were two more gifts: exquisite, impeccably hand-stitched kantha textiles. Very different from my Nanu's clean, straight stitches on her blankets. These were ornately stitched into a piece of art, nothing practical about its function. These were meant to be displayed, not forgotten in some trunk. When Ma revealed them to us, I started weeping. Seeing the little terracotta red and blue stitches, my Dadi's painstaking threadwork, for the first time, I felt her presence. Lutfunnessa, my ancestor, a great artist. For the past forty years, her descendants had not been curious enough to open that trunk.

Each intricate, complex, and beautiful stitch reminded me of the act of writing a book, word by word, sentence by sentence, until text is woven into textile. Each stitch is a testament to Dadi's concentration, her brilliant skill. The discovery of this heirloom, soon after I turned forty—for my Dadi, an age a few years shy of death—felt so significant. As a multidisciplinary artist, I try not to let the years of obscurity, of living in the work without rest, steal the joy of being on the journey. The ambition of reaching that point when you release the final work, along with the revelry after, has an addictive quality. It can't be our reason, but it's something we all work toward, it's what keeps us going, that another person might be moved by our work. Dadi made this textile for the beauty, the challenge, the flex. Holding this work, at this age, I feel the weight of this work, the weight of her pain. I wonder, when she made it, did she believe that she would live long enough to meet her son Bablu's children?

I rubbed my hands along the curved stitches made by her hand, a laying of hands, touching my foremother's art, where she embedded her genius, perhaps waiting for us to someday find it and finally meet her.

//

When I perfume, I work through borderless body language, sniffing each composition on skin, melding liquid materials meant to evaporate into the air. One of the aspects of perfume that's always called to me is the acute way in which our scent sense becomes activated when we remember our trauma. When we remember the notes of laundry, blood, fruit, fear. This remembering through the wordless is part of what has drawn me to scent. What comes after the ashes of war, genocide, pandemic, but beauty? The inviolable beauty of every human, animal, and ecosystem is what persists, beyond domination. During these past few strange years, I lost some of the deepest femme friendships I've known. *Lost* may be imprecise; in each of these relationships, I've had to examine my own role, as vanisher, as the one who went radio silent to tend to myself. The Ghost. So often, I turn women and femmes into my muse. What is the nature of a muse but to know that one day, her visitations are meant to cease?

Love between femmes is a powerful bond, but there are clashes that open a wound so deep in each other, and a potent rage, that being in each other's presence feels untenable. In each fracture, I played every role: Victim. Survivor. Perpetrator. Wrongdoer. Shit-talker. Bitch. In each fracture, I found it easier to let go of them than to swallow another's femme's feelings and suffocate my own in the process. In each fracture, the love morphed into distrust. Small, cold words hardly touching the magma beneath—

You've judged me. You made me feel like I was walking on eggshells. I'm taking space from you. You remind me of my abuser. You blew me off. You'd never do that to a white person. You disregarded me. You must really, really hate me. You're a narcissist.

Or—

Nothing.

Silence.

When I think back to these exchanges—all of which happened through the detached, inhuman medium of text or email—I wish I'd chosen warmth. My voice. My presence.

None of my excuses—depression after dozens of rejections from publishers, a yearlong bout of coronavirus, finishing a book—excuse my behavior. Like everyone, I've felt the constant exhaustion of swimming against the tide of the world—as these femme friends did, too. That life raft of us, which once tethered us, unraveled. It hurt. But it felt as necessary as burning land for new brush to grow. Femme love—nonsexual, nonblood—when it turns into femme loss, shatters a sacred, chosen sisterhood. What hurts more than losing the comforting voice of a friend you once cherished? I've swerved between alienation and romanticization. An act of mythmaking. Turning these femmes I once loved but can no longer bear to be around into potent memories, or nemeses. During the past half decade of experiencing strange parasocial relationships, enduring technologically induced isolation, and witnessing violence too cruel to be adequately described by language, I've come to understand that these femme fractures have forced me to evolve. These breakups forced me to reckon with toxic behavior that keeps me from liberation. Only another femme can pull you through that pain (or put you through it) with a profound rage and love. Only another femme can abandon you, shatter your heart, and force you to come back to your own wholeness. Becoming femme means you lay down your armor, your vulnerability as strong as your power; every adornment or ritual, every expression of joy or rage, is a luminous offering, a supernova indistinguishable from the unfurling of the Universe. *Femme*, moving toward chaos and destruction, *femme*, until the inevitable—rebirth.

LUSUS DEUX

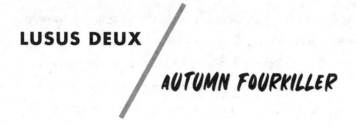

AUTUMN FOURKILLER

I am the three things a woman should never be.

A Sunday school teacher once said that the purity I kept long after others had shed theirs was a gift, that I must have been chosen for something, set aside. Now, I wonder what was so repulsive about me that she felt the need to comfort me in this way. And, of course, whether she knows anything of what I am.

//

The first kiss I truly remember (an important distinction) came to me in my sophomore year of college, and even then, I don't remember it well—I was too nervous, burning red, vision whiting out at the edges. It was barely a peck, soft lips against bitten ones. They said, "That was sweet." I said nothing—my voice dried up, my mouth deserted and tongue cottony.

Later, after I had left their car, and made my way back to my dorm to shiver and shake under mounds of blankets, I texted them, saying I can't do this, I couldn't see them again. It was too much for me, it was too much—

They were disappointed; I had seemed so perfect on paper, hadn't I? I was so funny, smart, so charming. The cracks I saw in the mirror weren't visible to the casual observer, and people frequently made me out to be a better person than I was. Some days I could barely recognize my own reflection, and though I didn't hate what I saw, I knew with clarity that no one could ever love me or my body—not in the way *normal* people got loved. I had made my peace with that. I had. There was nothing to be done.

That night, tears dripped into my thick, dark sideburns and I didn't wipe them. I let them soak into my skin and pretended I was at the bottom of a river, cocooned in wombsound and deep, dark water.

//

I knew that body hair fetish existed, especially on the internet, but I had no practical knowledge of it. It seemed like a fluke— *sure, they may love the hair, but what of the fat, what of the—*

I am too charming to be truly insufferable, which is why it makes no sense that I am alone and refuse to let anyone love me. I am fickle in that I worry about divorce despite never having been married. Finding someone obsessed with a singular part of me, still, seems like the only pathway to love.

Whoever might love my body, much less the spirit occupying it, must also be malformed. We would make a pair, in that way, wouldn't we?

//

It is more expedient to describe the places on my body where I do not have hair, or dark patches, than it is to try to list them all, but that is not what you're here for. You want the visceral, the monstrous. Let me give it to you.

The most disturbing to *the outside world* (not the microcosm that is my body, my blood, the people who love me, who choose me) must be the places that are supposed to mark me as female. My breasts, the space between them, my rounded, pendulous abdomen, my upper thighs, my buttocks, my face. The hair is black, thick, wiry, and pubic in its intensity—and my skin is white. When I was a child, I looked more Native than I do now. I was tanned by the sun; I had not yet sequestered myself away.

And—*What is looking Native anyway? What is—*

//

An early memory—one of my preschool classmates says I am too big and heavy to be on the merry-go-round with him and that I need to get off.

I probably cry, or, given trends later in my life, blush deeply and go silent and rigid.

I am an achingly lonely child and, yes, large. I can't help what I am. I can only try to make myself smaller by hunching my shoulders, and saying nothing, and taking up as little air as possible. The Bible says you are beautifully and wonderfully made. The Bible says you are an abomination, secretive, *you cannot hide from us, Little Girl, we will stretch out our hands and—*

No one can say I do not learn my lessons quickly.

//

You are wondering, and so I will sate your curiosity. I am the three things a woman should never be—fat, ugly (without curation), and hairy.

In this way, I am a born sinner. In this way, I am exactly what I am supposed to be.

//

Two months after my father dies, the hair on my head begins to fall out in clumps. At the time, I'm living in an old Mexican woman's attic in the suburbs of northern Alabama. My scalp is so pale it almost looks translucent, and it makes me vaguely nauseated to look at it for too long. I hear Fox News blaring from downstairs, and my hands don't shake when I reach for the craft scissors.

In some tribes, this kind of ritual is sacred. It isn't meant to be taken lightly.

And yet, all my elders are dead, or at least their bodies are dead. I am Cherokee by blood, Yuchi by practice.

I cut at least a foot of hair off and put it in a gallon Ziploc freezer bag for later review. I run my fingers through what is left and think, *I hope they can hide my bald spot in my coffin.*

//

The first time someone laughs *specifically* at the fur coating me from head to toe, I'm at Girl Scout camp.

I am still not sure how I was accepted, as I was too bashful for group activities and generally averse to anything that involved *putting myself out there.* My mother's best friend from college—my aunt █████—lets me spend the week with her, as the camp is an hour or so from my home and my mother works, at minimum, three jobs.

At the camp, we sing, hike through the woods, and pick Scout names. I don't remember what mine was, but I will imagine it was something along the lines of Coyote or Sparrow. Maybe Shadow.

The ringleader of our group—the Cowboys—is our camp counselor's daughter. She is petite and already beautiful in a way that *can* make middle schoolers mean. She has a friend from before, who is shorter and less beautiful, but still biting.

I am alone, with my book, on a bench, during one of the short breaks we get throughout the day. They come out of the cabin and start giggling. I can feel them staring at me in a way that makes my ears red, but I don't look up. Finally, one of them, I don't remember who, says, "Your legs are so hairy. Why don't you shave them? It's gross." Then, they burst into twin smirks, and for a moment, everything goes silent. I shake my head, or mumble something like, "I just—I don't—I—" I don't sob then, but I do later.

I stare at the ground for the rest of the day. I don't make conversation; I speak only to answer direct questions. When I get home, I ask my mother if she can help me, and she does, and nicks me only once.

I am nine years old. I am in third grade. My grandfather calls me Little Victoria, after my mother, and baby doll. The last time I saw my father he was drunk and mean, and it was only for a moment until we went away. I have paralyzing thoughts and strange urges to pray in circles, and sometimes I can't stop myself from imagining all the pains of hell, which I will surely go to, because I am a bad *girl* and I dress like a boy, and I am—

I do not get to be a child because I do not *look* like a child is supposed to look. I am thought to be ill-suited for innocence, for carnival rides, for softness.

My legs feel strange, not quite silky. They make me feel sick to my stomach in a way I will not realize for years is anxiety—clinical, and severely so.

I don't wear shorts in public for another decade.

//

When I am five years old, my bone age is that of a twenty-year-old. I grow six inches in six months and gain weight the moment food enters my mouth. My mother takes me to an endocrinologist in Tulsa, Oklahoma. His name is Dr. ███, and he scares me. I cry when he looks at my privates. He does some blood work. He says I will eventually even out, at least in height, and in that, at least, he is right. He's brisk and answers my mother's questions, but not nicely. No one explains anything to me; no one even offers.

In all other doctors' offices, in all other lives, I will not cry, but I will want to. They will say, "Time to lose some weight." When I say I can't, I will see their barely contained eye rolls. They will look at my vagina and breasts, which no one has ever seen outside a clinical context. They will change the diagnoses. They will not have any answers for me because it is a woman's disease, and no one cares about women's diseases. I will never have children. I will not burden a child with my brain, my body. I say as much, but I get tongue clicks, shaken heads. I am not to be trusted with my body. I have ruined it, with my dark red stretch marks and mustache and wanting to die.

If only, if only.

//

Polycystic ovary syndrome. Benign adrenal tumors. Adult-onset adrenal hyperplasia. None of these things; all of them. Heightened cortisol levels. Excess testosterone. Not trying hard enough. Insulin resistance. Gluttony. Genetics. Nothing conclusive. All in your head. No research. Why are you so afraid? What the fuck is wrong with you?

//

I take a memory and cross it out.

I give an embroidery artist three nude photographs of me spread-eagle on the country house's floor—the prompt is gender euphoria. "Don't worry," they say. "This won't hurt a bit."

When I was a child, I hoped I would get breast cancer and they'd have to take it all and then everyone would pity, not hate, me. I was horrible.

"I only liked to be fucked here," I say, pointing. "But pretend it's another place." I don't actually care if it's another place, but the lie helps. The man who likes my body hair and how many times I can orgasm in a row but does not care for my conception of a gender says, "Yes, yes, anything."

My leg hair looks how I believe it should look. Though there is a weird empty patch on my right ankle from where I once tried to wax to make my mother happy.

//

In my second year of graduate school, I download an app marketed toward threesomes. I am bored, and lonely, and want some attention. I select all the best pictures of myself and add a bio that makes me seem like less of an in-between thing, more ghost than *girl.* I match with a couple, both ginger, who say that "body hair is a turn-on." After a lackluster entry, they ask for pictures—but not nudes. They want to see my armpits, my bare legs, the skin near my wrists, my knuckles. I send them, more confused than anything, and not particularly worried about what is going to happen. While they aren't artful, they aren't mundane. I wait for a response, wondering if I have made a mistake but—what are they going to do? Sell them? I don't care enough to continue to interrogate the thought.

I clean my desk off, I vacuum, I watch TikToks, I take my vitamins, I wait.

Then, a storm. Emojis—hearts, tongues, beads of sweat. Peaches and eggplants. Lips, clapping hands. Shocked eyes.

They say, "You're the hottest person we've ever seen."

They say, "We're so turned on."

They say, "I am so hard. I am so wet. I want your mouth. Your hands. Your ass. Your ███."

They say, "How can you be real?"

They say—

//

Later, the man asks me if I want to watch him edge himself. I am sitting eating cantaloupe with chopsticks and writing. "Maybe later," I write, knowing I will never, ever do that.

Later, I delete the app, having gotten what I wanted, but I am hot, flushed. I am no longer a child, a terrified teenager. I have come into a political and social awareness, an anticolonized consciousness. I refuse to think of myself in the terms of those who have no understanding, no emotional intelligence. I am loved, I have many good friends. I am moderately successful, an early career writer. I have one foot stuck on the other side, I—

And yet—once again I am reduced. I am flustered by attention and *apparent attraction*. I am afraid of my own freedom. I am afraid of what happens when I accept what I am.

And—*what am I?*

//

In my dreams, my body resists change. There is no transformation, no chrysalis.

In my daydreams, the person who is meant for me must love, does love, the things I dislike about my body, the handfuls of it. How big my chest is, the ████████, the way I enjoy penetration when I feel like I should not, my need to be reclined.

And I got a late start to physicality, but what I lost in time I made up for in inventiveness.

And it's true that I tire quickly of games that are not of my own design, the ones I know all the rules to. I dislike being teased.

And I am probably obsessed with God, but not in the way anyone who loved me as a child would be proud of.

And in my dreams, I have two partners. What does it say about me that I feel the force of myself, of my body, must be spread out?

And in the not-so-hidden caverns of my heart I crave money and power and recognition. I crave it all.

There, there. The flesh is weak, yet the spirit is oh, oh, so willing.

COMING TO LIGHT

ALL POWER TO THE PEOPLE

RAQUEL WILLIS

There is no pride without protest.

ALL POWER TO THE PEOPLE.
ALL POWER TO THE PEOPLE.
ALL POWER TO THE PEOPLE.

With mellifluous bombast, activist Qween Jean chanted these words and riled up a hundreds-deep rally crowd at Brooklyn's Grand Army Plaza. With these words, she channeled an essential Diana Davies portrait of queer movement forebear Marsha P. Johnson. In it, Johnson holds a minimal white sign with the war cry written in thin black lettering. It was a necessary reminder on this oppressive day in June 2024 that the energy of our most radical social justice forebears coursed through us. I watched as this young leader, who represented a new generation, claimed her power.

On more than one occasion, Qween had shared that my speech

at the Brooklyn Liberation March almost exactly four years earlier had served as a wake-up call for her. In it, I declared, "I believe in Black trans power," conducting a crowd of nearly twenty thousand to pledge the same. I felt honored that I'd played a part in her journey, and it was then that I truly started to see myself as delivering on a commitment to collective liberation that I'd made a decade before.

I'd stumbled into activism after the untimely deaths by suicide of two young teens, Leelah Alcorn and Blake Brockington, in the months when 2014 blended into 2015. The former was just seventeen years old when she published a letter on social media that revealed how she didn't see a future for herself as a trans adult. She'd been driven to her final act after being forced into conversion therapy by her ultra-Christian parents. Brockington's life transformed after he became the first openly trans high school homecoming royal in North Carolina. His win sparked intense media scrutiny, but it didn't deter him from using the attention to organize in his local community and speak out against anti-Black police brutality and transphobia. Unfortunately, in time, his longstanding depression would steer him toward the end of his life.

I absorbed their stories, yearning to make sense of why the world seemed so determined to make trans people, especially youth, feel so insignificant. It made sense that the world seemed uninhabitable to Blake and Leelah. I felt lucky that I'd somehow survived adolescence despite growing up in a traditionally Southern, devoutly Catholic family. Sometimes I consider it a blessing that I didn't understand my full truth as a trans woman until I was at the edge of adulthood in college. While my high school years weren't always smooth as an openly gay student, I was shielded from the inevitably more difficult experience of being openly trans at such a young age in the first decade of the twenty-first century.

I was around twenty-one when I embarked on my gender transition. At the University of Georgia, I delved into queer student activism and found community, largely made up of non-Black transmasculine folks and cis lesbians. I was isolated from other Black trans people, as there weren't many attending the school or living openly in the surrounding local area. But I cobbled together whatever information I could find about the trans experience from forums and word of mouth. In the year leading up to my graduation, I had a sound plan for starting hormone replacement therapy, updating my identity documents, and crossing that final stage to grab my journalism degree presenting as my truest self.

While the collegiate environment had mostly shielded me from bigotry and discrimination, I knew to be out at my first place of employment would be a gamble. Sure, more trans people were showing up in the media. Figures like actress Laverne Cox and author (now television writer and producer) Janet Mock gave me hope for a brighter future. But all that visibility hadn't quite touched small-town Georgia. So, I held my identity close. In fact, I only came out to a few people in my first job as a reporter at a local newspaper, and only after I sensed I could trust them. Both were co-workers. One was a cisgender, bisexual Black woman I clocked after she used gender-neutral pronouns to refer to her female partner. The other was a sweet, older white woman who confided in me that she had a daughter who was a lesbian. While they gave me some reprieve from that mostly conservative environment, I eventually moved to Atlanta and found another job working in digital publishing.

In my first few months there, I kept quiet about my truth, pledging only to divulge more to my co-workers if ever specifically prompted about my identity. But the deaths of Alcorn and Brockington shattered any illusion that there was glory in hiding my truth. I felt complicit in their demises, so I spoke up online. In the mid-2010s, it was still fairly novel for everyday trans people to be outspoken about discrimination and violence on social media. So, I garnered a following and a bit of acclaim. Outside of my day job, I was a freelance writer. After an essay I wrote about dating as a Black transgender woman went viral, Cox amplified it. A local reporter, Darian Aaron, picked up the fact that she had given me a call-out. And that was the first time I saw myself referred to as an activist in the media.

Beyond my growing visibility, my most formative experiences came when I started organizing in the Atlanta social justice scene. I applied for an internship with Solutions Not Punishments Coalition (now Collaborative) and met Toni-Michelle Williams, who led the program. I learned about the ills of criminalization and police profiling, particularly as it pertains to trans and gender-nonconforming people as well as sex workers. As an intern, I was simply chasing my passion for the well-being and progress of our community. I never would have envisioned just how valuable my voice would become to our movement.

Yet, here I was in New York City, part of a lineup of formidable speakers. Our goal was to sound the alarm on an upcoming city budget vote that promised to cut funds from schools ($100M), nurses ($65M), libraries ($58M), parks ($55M), museums ($26.3M), and HIV/AIDs programs ($5.3M) in service of Mayor Eric Adams's disastrous agenda to expand policing and prisons.

If you were in that audience, it's likely you learned about the event from a scarlet digital flyer reading "NOT GAY AS IN HAPPY, QUEER AS IN F**K ERIC ADAMS." Adding to the provocation was a grayscale cutout of the New York City mayor's head, marred with asterisk-like symbols over his eyes.

This rally served as a debut for Gender Liberation Movement (GLM), a new collective I'd had the pleasure of creating with other organizers after the success of two massive marches in Brooklyn during the summers of 2020 and 2021. While those efforts had focused on Black trans lives and trans youth, respectively, we became interested in building a larger coalition to mobilize against all kinds of gender-based sociopolitical threats. We saw the rally as an opportunity to debut GLM's mission of responding through media, direct action, and policy. We knew that continued police brutality and expansion of the prison industrial complex at the expense of more generative and necessary social services sat at the heart of our fight.

Many of the activists, organizers, and concerned community members who made it out to the plaza near an ovoid roadway were still making sense of the past four years. Vehicles rushed past, a reminder of the vast majority of folks simply living, trying to ignore all that we'd collectively endured. There was the world-altering COVID-19 pandemic, the broadcast police murder of George Floyd, a historic summer of protest, a backlash toward activist demands for defunding police and prisons, and a presidential swap from ultranationalist Republican Donald Trump to chronically centrist Joseph Biden. While easily impressed Democrats celebrated the supposed return of pre-Trump "status quo" political leadership, a backlash, fueled mainly by liberal qualms about "too-leftist" messaging, fed the expansion of the carceral system.

According to *Policing Progress*, a 2024 American Civil Liberties Union report,* while LGBTQ+ people experience more police-initiated contact than non-LGBTQ+ people, transgender people are searched significantly more than our cisgender LGBQ+ counterparts. And Black trans people were the most likely to have experienced physical force by the police among all LGBTQ+ people by race.

Although the criminalization of trans people is openly discussed more than it probably ever has been, the US has long demonized those who transcend gender norms. Some of our earliest records of trans existence come in the form of court documents. For instance, in 1836, Mary Jones** was put on trial in court and the media as a person assigned male at birth who navigated the world as a woman. Allegedly, she stole a john's wallet while engaging in sex work. But the papers at the time made a spectacle out of her identity. We can see a throughline from that coverage in the nineteenth century to the ongoing struggles that trans people face now.

In the 2024 US elections, Republicans spent nearly $215 mil-

---

* Jordan Grasso, Stefan Vogler, Emily Greytak, Casey Kindall, and Valerie Jenness, *Policing Progress: Findings from a National Survey of LGBTQ+ People's Experiences with Law Enforcement* (American Civil Liberties Union, 2024).
** C. R. Snorton, *Black on Both Sides: A Racial History of Trans Identity* (University of Minnesota Press, 2017).

lion on ads demonizing trans people, particularly those who are incarcerated or detained.

Organizers in the GLM network and our partners with The People's Plan didn't need a report to tell us this. In fact, many of us had been working on abolition and decriminalization efforts for years—from defending sex work to ending cash bail and solitary confinement. My fellow GLM cofounder and friend, Eliel Cruz, and I deepened our bond while doing media strategy to elevate the life and story of twenty-seven-year-old Layleen Polanco.* Polanco, an Afro-Latina trans woman, died in state custody at the infamous Rikers Island in 2019.

Layleen's death, just weeks before the fiftieth anniversary of the Stonewall Uprising, signaled just how much the initial fight of our movement, spurred by our ancestors and transcestors, had been deprioritized. While capitalism and corporatism had focused singularly on the air of celebration ushered in by Christopher Street Liberation Day observances of the 1970s, over time, they fully obscured the radical and militant elements of that seminal series of events, long considered the birth of the modern LGBTQ+ rights movement.

That uprising, as I often remind folks, is rooted in the fight against police brutality and profiling and the incarceration of folks on the margins. Many a Stonewall Riots witness will tell you that Black and brown queens (further described as trans, drag, street, scare, and otherwise) were key to ushering in a culture of defiance of norms instead of capitulation to them. GLM

---

* Raquel Willis, "Layleen Cubilette-Polanco Died in the System, but Her Fight Lives On," *Out*, June 2019.

wanted to deliver a counterpoint to the mainstream observances of Pride Month, something that harkened to the community's, or at least the movement's, more radical roots. Our organizers saw holding the criminal (in)justice system accountable and calling for abolition as a mandate bequeathed to us from queer and trans ancestors. And Adams seemed like the perfect culprit to critique.

Since his ascension from Brooklyn Borough president to mayor, he'd exalted the efforts of law enforcement above nearly anything else. His allegiance to the carceral system was something he wore, quite literally, like a badge of honor—inspired by his stints as an officer with the New York Police Department (NYPD) and the New York City Transit Police. Of course, we opposed his leadership. After all, he was an extension of the very entity and system that our ancestors and transcestors had opposed at the start of the LGBTQIA+ movement.

Our collective was so unimpressed by Adams's resume that we drafted a more fitting one in the caption for the rally flyer, urging would-be attendees to "REJECT THE LOOMING FASCISM OF LITERAL BATMAN VILLAIN ERIC ADAM$ AND HI$ ENABLER$' CORRUPT, CAPITALIST, QUEERPHOBIC, SEROPHOBIC, WHORE-PHOBIC, ANTI-POOR, ANTI-PROTEST, ANTI-NIGHTLIFE, ANTI-ART, ANTI-ELDER, ANTI-ACTIVIST, ANTI-EDUCATION POLICE-STATE."

Our promotional bluster, however justified, didn't do justice to the community care that went into the planning of the action. Photographers Hunter Abrams and Stas Ginzburg, no strangers to covering our rallies, lovingly documented the presence of respected speakers and leaders such as wisecracking, forever glam Ceyenne Doroshow, founder of Gays and Lesbians Living in a Transgender Society (GLITS, Inc.). The sweltering sun was no match for our safety team, which monitored the disbursement of water and sunscreen to rallygoers. This kind of care and loving power was an antidote to Adams's agenda.

//

Shortly after Qween Jean retired her black bullhorn, Ianne Fields Stewart and Fran Tirado took to microphone stands on scrappy staging. Like me, they had delved into the unspoken uniform of the day: tank-top silhouettes, pink armbands designating our connection to the event's organizing team, and "ready-to-work" high ponytails.

As they welcomed the crowd to the official program, my eyes scanned the crowd. We were surrounded by crimson, triangular banners with slogans like "CARE NOT COPS," "NYPL NOT NYPD," and "LESS JAILS MORE WHORES." After taking them in, I focused on the first few speakers. Zara Nasir, executive director of The People's Plan NYC, discussed how Adams had averaged two budget cuts annually since taking office three years earlier. She mentioned the People's Budget Campaign's demands,* which included investing in public infrastructure with union labor, essential services like public education and social safety nets, and divesting from criminalization and budgetary waste.

Just after Nasir finished, Jawanza James Williams, the director of organizing for Voices of Community Activists and Leaders (VOCAL-NY), led a poetic call to ancestors. The crowd hushed

---

* "2024 People's Budget Campaign," The People's Plan NYC, accessed January 7, 2025.

as his valorous words washed over us: "I hear the voices of centuries past. Singing in chorus a language my tongue will never speak. But I feel it deep in my bones when Black queer blood wets the earth. And another opens their mouth. From which crawls the parts of revolution. Words for some, movements for others, but all of them demanding dignity. Asé."

Following a reverent pause, he shared the story of Kawaski Trawick, a thirty-two-year-old Black gay man killed by the NYPD in 2019. Remembered as a gifted dancer and a personal trainer, at the time, Trawick was living in supportive housing in the Bronx. After barging into his apartment, two officers refused to answer his questions about why they were in his home.

This is how a *ProPublica* investigative report described the altercation: "Instead of trying to ease the confrontation, the officers escalated it. They ordered Trawick to drop the knife. They ignored his repeated questions about why they were there. And then one of the officers took it further. First he used his Taser on Trawick, despite his more-experienced partner telling him not to. When Trawick became enraged, the younger officer, who is white, fired his gun, despite his partner, who is Black, again trying to stop him."*

Trawick's demise, not unlike Polanco's, broke through the hypothetical harms previously mentioned in the space. They made clear the precarity of our lives in a city that continuously sees folks on the margins—be they queer, trans, Black, brown, disabled, or poor—as a problem.

---

* Eric Umansky, "It Wasn't the First Time the NYPD Killed Someone in Crisis. For Kawaski Trawick, It Only Took 112 Seconds," *ProPublica*, December 4, 2020.

NO JUSTICE, NO PEACE.

NO JUSTICE, NO PEACE.

INVEST IN HEALTHCARE NOT POLICE.

INVEST IN HEALTHCARE NOT POLICE.

Ariel Friedlander, one of the core organizers of the rally, led off with a chant before sharing her speech. As a Jewish, anti-Zionist leader, she'd worked alongside other members of Jewish Voices for Peace and ACT-UP for months on pro-Palestinian and antigenocide efforts. As she spoke about the connection between abolitionist and antiwar mobilizations, the crowd roared. Interspersed between trans and Progress Pride flags were countless Palestinian flags and folks adorned in kaffiyehs, nodding to the almost yearlong heightened organizing in response to Israel's genocidal onslaught on Gaza. Moreover, another gripe about the NYPD was its heavy participation in the law enforcement exchange programs between the United States and Israel. *Deadly Exchange*, a 2018 report published by Jewish Voices for Peace and Researching the American-Israeli Alliance, explains how this decades-long relationship fosters an expansion in surveillance, justification for racial profiling, and the forcible suppression of public protests not too dissimilar from the one in which we were engaged.

Many of us had been browbeaten over our support for Palestinians in the months prior. A common line of thought from Zionists was that Israel was a bastion of queer equality while the predominantly Arab and Muslim populations of the Middle East represented a threat to our existence. But we knew better, and we knew that Adams's allegiance to Israeli Prime Minister Benjamin Netanyahu served as another reason to denounce his plans.

The bold declarations for a "Free Palestine" melted into applause for movement-lawyer-turned-political-commentator Olayemi Olurin. Over the past year, she'd made a name for herself through viral videos and clips, some of which exposed the most glaring misdeeds of the Adams administration. Her crowning moment as Adams's "No. 1 Hater" occurred during a debate on the morning radio show *The Breakfast Club*. While going toe-to-toe with the mayor on his record, she left him undeniably shook for the world to see. At this rally, she didn't let up on her crusade. In fact, in the conclusion of her speech, she declared, "Eric Adams is an enemy of the people. He is an enemy of progress. And we need to make him a one-time mayor."

As speakers came, inspired, and went, my time at the mic inched closer. Generally, I trust that the words to move the crowd will come. Rarely have I let myself down on that account. Still, the nerves were there. Of all of the experiences, years of memories, and knowledge of our collective histories swirling within my mind—which ones would my voice bring to the fore?

I'd been reflecting on my relationship to abolition in the days leading up to the rally. Like most others, my introduction to the concept was through scattered grade-school lessons about enslavement and the Civil War. It seemed to be terminology forever crystallized in the 1800s with figures like Frederick Douglass and Sojourner Truth. I'd coursed all through adolescence and college without any deeper thought about the prison industrial complex. That was largely reflective of my privilege—all that middle-class, respectable mumbo jumbo within which I grew up.

Like many other Black folks, I had also grown up with a healthy distrust of the police. I'd heard the mantra "don't trust the popo" for as long as I could remember. And, of course, I'd absorbed images in history books of white law enforcement hosing down and siccing dogs on civil rights movement protesters. And while I knew there were myriad ways for a Black person to get swallowed up by America's criminal (in)justice system, I had also been indoctrinated with damaging and dehumanizing ideas about people who had been arrested and incarcerated. My Grandma Inez said to all her grandkids, "If I ever get a call that you're in jail, I'm telling them to keep you in there until you get some goddamn sense." It was implied that those caught up in the system were disposable and must have been doing something wrong to warrant such treatment, and we fully adopted this thinking as young people. It was community organizing in 2010s Atlanta that changed that for me. So, that's what I decided to focus on and, lo and behold, our Cop City fight in New York was all intertwined with the recent fights regarding Atlanta's Cop City as well.

After some last-minute processing of the words of the previous speakers and deep breaths, I took the stage to address the crowd.

It's hot out here, right? But we know this heat, this political wildfire we're facing right now, is nothing compared to what our family around the globe is facing. All of our family facing genocide, right? Our Palestinian family, our Sudanese family, our Congolese family, and all of our family facing genocide, facing erasure. Our Indigenous family facing erasure around the globe.

We're here because we know that to be invested in police and policing, to be invested in prisons, is to be invested in death. And we are not invested in death. Are we? We are demanding that our leaders divest from death and invest in lives.

Invest in Black lives, invest in Black trans lives, invest in poor lives, invest in homeless lives, houseless lives, Palestinian lives.

And divest. So I'm from Augusta, Georgia, but I cut my teeth community organizing in Atlanta. So this "Cop City" shit is real personal to me because we know that what we're facing right here is connected to what's happening nationally. We know that we're not facing the only Cop City, right? We know that there are Cop Cities that are all across this nation, and they're planning more. They're beefing them up, right? So when we fight against Queens' Cop City, we're fighting against all Cop Cities, right?

In Atlanta, I was working with my political home, Solutions Not Punishment Collaborative, with my dear friend Toni-Michelle Williams. This was back in 2015, 2016. And we worked on a report because we knew that queer and trans folks, especially Black queer and trans folks, especially Black trans women, especially Black trans sex workers, are disproportionately impacted by policing.

And the name of our report was the most dangerous thing out here. The most dangerous thing out here is the police. So, can y'all say that the most dangerous thing out here is the police? Fuck them cops.

And so I know down in Atlanta, one of the people on the front lines, our dear nonbinary, Indigenous sibling, Tortuguita, was shot. At least fourteen times by state troopers for protesting, just like we are today. Because we know that the most dangerous thing out here is what? It is what? The police. And so we don't believe in police power.

Fuck police power. We believe in people power, right? So can you say it? Fuck police power? We believe in people power.

So it makes sense, right, that we are gathering about a week out, not even, from the anniversary of the Stonewall Riots. And if you don't know, you better fucking know that that was a queer militant uprising against the NYPD. There is no pride in genocide, and there is no pride without protest.

There is no pride in genocide. There is no pride without protest.

So remember when you think about our figures, right? Stormé, Marsha, Sylvia, Zazu Nova, another erased Black icon. And so many others. They were protesting against the NYPD. So I don't want to hear anything about queer and trans liberation unless you understand that we have a birthright to protest the police.

And we have a mandate to protest the police. We have a mandate to divest from death. And invest in lives, divest from death, invest in lives. So we need our leaders. And it ain't many leaders we can call on today, right? It's not enough leaders that have called for a ceasefire. It's not. They so scared. There aren't enough that believe in Palestinian lives.

It's not enough to actually believe in Black lives. It's not enough to actually believe in queer and trans lives, and on and on. But we're demanding that our council believe in these lives, right? So we want that vote to represent what the people want. And the people want you to divest from death and invest in lives.

Divest from death. Invest in lives. Thank you.

Soon after I left the platform, Ceyenne Doroshow, ever the grande dame, stunned the audience with her presence as the final speaker. In a year in which our community had lost the great Cecilia Gentili, the preciousness of our elders became all the more clear. If anyone present most represented the mandate from our Stonewall ancestors, it was Ceyenne Doroshow.

She explained her dream of GLITS owning property to support the community in flourishing. To her, that was the antidote to the ever-expanding carceral system. It would be a refuge for all of the queer and trans folks, the Black and brown folks, and, as she said, the "whores who take care of the community." As she reminded us of her vision, she shone a light on the generative element of abolition. It's not solely about tearing down and ending what exists or even eviscerating the villains like Adams, who constantly try to shrink our lives. It's also about what we can build and create, especially through sacred queerness, that can serve the collective.

GENDER EUPHORIA IS A POWER SOURCE

CARO DE ROBERTIS

A power source can be a nourishment.
It can also be a powder keg.

In October of 2022, I visited the TransLatin@ Coalition office to interview Bamby Salcedo, the founder and executive director, for an oral history project. Bamby is a trans community icon and an extraordinarily busy person, so I'd arrived early, intent on making the best of every minute. She'd carved out two hours for me, no more, no less. And yet, when she came to the lobby to welcome me—exuding warmth and a quiet, graceful power—she would not sit for the interview until she'd introduced me to every staff member in the office that day. As I responded to each warm introduction, in Spanish, my tongue stumbled, stretched to make new shapes. With every *pleasure to meet you* I gendered myself, revealed myself, exposed.

This wasn't my first time speaking Spanish since my pronoun

transition, but it was my first time doing so in a trans Latinx space. I did not anticipate what it would open in me.

In English, gendered language is generally conferred on us by people when they talk about us to others—"They live next door"; "that's her car." Pronouns are something we tell others about, so they can speak of us respectfully in ways that mirror or reflect who we are. Of course, this happens in other languages too. But in Spanish, we also constantly gender ourselves, inflecting our adjectives with the masculine *o*, the feminine *a*, or the recently innovated gender-neutral *e* (or *x* in some US Latinx spaces). You cannot say you are tired, excited, or angry without gendering that experience. When you are pleased to meet someone, you are *encantado, encantade,* or *encantada.*

Though I'd been using they/them pronouns for about a year, I'd recently experimented with all pronouns (an approach that held authenticity for me but that I soon abandoned for cis-dominated spaces because of how often people, bewildered and seeing an AFAB person, reverted to she/her). Here, at the TransLatin@ Coalition, gendering my joy at meeting these trans women, I was mostly encantado and encantade, with a few encantadas slipping in. A blend, a mix, a male and female swirl. How would that land? Was I enough? Was I just confusing? That old fear arose, of being too strange or of adhering insufficiently to the framework of what I said I was, the framework I longed to call my home. It took me until my midforties to come out fully as genderqueer, then also as trans, not because I didn't know my inner landscape, but because my true gender is so fluid, so expansive, that I wasn't sure I had the right to claim the space. My gender would never be a settled thing, would never land tidily on one side of the binary and fold its limbs. I came of age and came out in the '90s, in a different iteration of queer culture when categories were more fixed. So that even now, that old fear flickered of being seen as illegible or as an interloper.

But it was only a flicker, and only in my own mind. As far as I knew, nobody in this trans space was imposing such narratives on me, except me. The TransLatin@ Coalition headquarters are warm, with colorful walls and the perpetual hum and bustle of radical community work, and I felt completely embraced by each office worker and by the environment as a whole. And however ordinary a pleasantry such as *pleased to meet you* may seem, with each exchange I felt the quiet thrill of speaking myself into being.

In Spanish, saying even the most ordinary things about myself can spark gender euphoria.

//

Gender euphoria—the joy or satisfaction of expressing or inhabiting one's full gender—is what lit my path to myself and made me whole. It's the glimmering thread I followed toward my own liberation. I didn't see myself as dysphoric, which is part of why it took me so long to recognize what I was; it was only after I tapped into the euphoria of living my whole gender that I understood that I'd been slightly dissociated from my body before, not in conscious pain, but also not entirely present. How could I have known what it was like to be fully embodied and awake? How could I have imagined the elation? When I leaned into my masculinity in a free and unapologetic way, cheerfully blending it with the rest of me, with nothing to prove to anyone, affirming the man in me without living as a man, existing, as the singer LP once put it, as a "tornado of male and female"—then suddenly I was keenly alive, and inhabiting my body and soul as never before.

I was completely unprepared for how I felt. How much energy was released, the pure vitality and ecstatic joy of being whole.

//

In her seminal essay "Uses of the Erotic: The Erotic as Power," Audre Lorde explores the erotic as a life force capable of fueling and fortifying us as, in her words, "a considered source of power and information in our lives." She points out that the erotic has been "vilified, abused, and devalued" in society, and calls on us to reclaim it as a "well of replenishing and provocative force" for our fulfillment, creative work, and contributions toward a better future for our communities.

Lorde originally presented these visionary ideas as a paper in 1978. At that time, she was specifically addressing women and, more particularly, lesbians and lesbians of color. I first read this essay in 1994, the spring I first came out, and have carried it inside me for over thirty years. Like many dykes, I've turned to it continuously as a touchstone, a foundational sacred text. Now, as I reflect on gender euphoria—its force, its potential—I find, in Lorde, a framework for understanding this unleashed joy not only as its own wonder, but as a deeper wellspring.

Lorde understood the connections between our embodied pleasure and the radical defiance of inhuman systems. She taught us that deepest inner truths are subversive and hold a vibrant capacity to nourish and sustain us if we let them.

Gender euphoria is an incredible feeling; it's also a power source.

To be clear, erotic energy and trans identity are not the same thing. They should not be conflated, especially since trans people's experiences are all too often reduced to our genitalia or to cis people's projections of hypersexuality. Our bodies do not exist only for sex or in sexual space, any more or less than other human bodies. We exist for ourselves. The thrill of being our full true gender is not always inherently erotic. And though gender euphoria can be entwined with the erotic—for example, when it arises with a lover who sees and feels and relishes your body in the ways you know it, that is an experience beyond compare—the two are distinct channels.

Nevertheless, we might think of the erotic and gender euphoria as parallel wellsprings of power, to which we have access as trans and gender-nonconforming people. Like overlapping circles in a Venn diagram, they are not the same but share some elements in common: both involve a fierce capacity for joy; both are reviled by the dominant culture; both have the potential to unleash in us the fuel to make our lives, in Lorde's words, "richer and more possible."

//

A power source can be a nourishment. It can also be a powder keg.

I thought my gender journey would be healing. And it was. It is. But also, a few months in, my marriage of twenty years collapsed. It did so spectacularly, at breathtaking speed, like a glacier whose fractures had gone hidden even to itself. It was a marriage that had begun in 2002, when unions like ours weren't legal anywhere in the country. I'd thought of our marriage as a kind of queer haven, which held particular meaning both culturally, as same-sex marriage rights became a battlefield around us, and personally, as I'd been disowned by my family of origin when I came out.

It would be overly simplistic to say that my gender transition caused the divorce. That is not the case. But it would also be false to call the timing a coincidence.

For some of us, the training to keep ourselves small or distort our own truth for the comfort of others runs deep, below consciousness. For those assigned female at birth, or for those raised by a malignant narcissist—as I was—we do it to ourselves at such a deep level that it goes unseen, even to us. We know what to do to keep the peace: Absorb blame. Placate. Shrink yourself. None of that worked as well once I let my whole gender exist in my skin. The change expanded me. It made me more vast inside than I'd quite known it was possible to be. All people of all genders are vast inside, of course, even if some of us have part of our life force buried under floorboards in the basements of our psyches. Gender euphoria ripped the floorboards out, freed the masculine in me. I had access to more of myself than ever before. Connected to my own truth, ecstatically alive, I became terrible at self-erasure. Any structure that relied on it was doomed.

As my marriage exploded, I leaned into the wind. I didn't know where I was going, but I trusted the journey—that however uncharted it might be, it would be true.

//

In the thick of that moment, when everything about my life was destabilized—my housing, my day-to-day parenting, my community, my trust, my financial survival, the maps of my potential futures—I began interviewing queer and trans BIPOC elders. I was fortunate enough to have a Baldwin-Emerson Fellowship, with a project called *I See My Light Shining* led by author and MacArthur Fellow Jacqueline Woodson. My assignment was to gather the oral histories of queer and trans elders of color of the West Coast, communities where I had deep networks and chosen family ties. I received training from the faculty at the Columbia University Center for Oral History Research, and state-of-the-art recording equipment that I hauled with me into the living rooms, kitchens, and offices of the remarkable elders who were kind enough to open their lives to me and share their voices and stories. The majority of the people I interviewed were gender-nonconforming: trans, nonbinary, genderqueer, transmasculine, transfeminine, gender-fluid, butch, and two-spirit people of color who'd paved the way for the freedoms and movements we know today.

Interviewing these people, and bearing witness to their stories, was one of the greatest honors of my life. It was also transformative. Later, their voices would be housed in an online archive, and I'd weave them into a book, but for now the experience was intimate. There I sat, microphone out, headphones on, listening deeply. Astounded. Blown away. Their voices are about so much more than me; still, in them, my torn-open soul found a continuous salve. *Here is a tale of survival. Of joy. Of the cost and power of stepping fully into your truth. Of what it took, and what it might take again, to be free. Of how I rose up. Of how I became. Of what community can mean. Of how we fought. Of how we shine.*

//

I asked each trans or gender-nonconforming narrator to share an early memory of gender euphoria—a time when, as a child, they experienced joy in their real gender. Some of the elders paused, having never been asked this question before. I watched some of their faces light up as they reached into memory for such a moment, pulling it up to be heard. Every single one of them had grown up in an environment where no adequate language existed for who they really were. And every single one of them had a gender euphoria story to tell.

Tina Valentín Aguirre, a Chicanx genderqueer and trans artist, activist, and cherished community leader, shared their experience seeing a Black trans woman walk past their elementary school fence every day. The woman spoke to young Tina, who felt a connection despite teachers' warnings to stay away. Tina felt seen by the woman, recognized as, in their own words, "a baby queer trans person," and affirmed in who they were. "That was the first time I had a euphoria, a joy, about gender."

Fresh "Lev" White, an activist, coach, teacher, and Black trans man, described the happiness he knew when he was free to play rough outside and come home with his clothes ripped and stained, the way boys did. "I can just feel it now," he said, "the excitement, the butterflies—not fear, but more like freedom. Yeah. I felt big." Sitting across from me in a Berkeley backyard, he extended his arms wide. "I'm just opening my arms to say, I felt big, and open, and fully available to be me."

As for accounts of gender euphoria later in life, they poured out generously. From the joys of intimacy or transition to drag adventures or bold acts of resistance, the power of trans euphoric life force was everywhere. Sharyn Grayson, a trailblazing activist and leader born in 1949, shared indelible memories of living openly as a young Black trans woman in the early 1970s. "I was like a person experiencing Rome or Italy for the first time, and you've always wanted to go," she said. "The clothes, the music, the environments, just walking down the street with friends, and guys flirting . . . Everything was wonderful about it. Oh, my God. I had so much fun. I was free. I was myself."

//

To be free in a world that seeks to cage us, we need new ways of speaking, new language for what we know. For me, the experience of gender euphoria is untranslatable, beyond words. And yet, I try. I fling metaphors around, flouting the rules, refusing to stick to a single image for something so vast. Gender euphoria as elixir. As flame. As descent: a musky plunge into earth, its lush darkness catching us, absorbing all light. Gender euphoria as light, piercing us with unsung joy as we lace those wingtips or don those earrings that are just right. Gender euphoria as nest, but also as flight, a tilt into the wind. Or as the wind itself, uplifting us, holding us aloft.

In my new chapter, I'm not just happier than before. I'm happy in ways I hadn't known were possible. Sometimes, gender euphoria moves through me with such strength that I feel as if I could live on that power source alone.

I can't, of course. We need more, much more, than euphoria for our individual and collective survival. But what might we be able to forge—what life, what breath, what cultural change—

when fueled by a joy so sharp it breaks through clouds, so deep we cannot help but call it home?

//

"We are shape-shifters," Tupili Lea Arellano, a two-spirit, trans, and butch Indigenous Chicanx activist and artist, said in their interview. "Performing in drag, I was euphoric. There's a power that comes with that, a hidden power we carry as two-spirit people, as people on the trans spectrum . . . That's a medicine. It's very powerful if we know how to use it."

//

I believe that Bamby Salcedo is pointing us in this same direction as Arellano, as Audre Lorde, when she urges us to "own our *jotería*." In preparation for my interview with Bamby at the TransLatin@ Coalition office, I watched videos of her giving speeches online, at rallies for trans justice, political protests, and community events. She speaks with tremendous passion, through megaphones, into microphones, unabashedly and radiantly loud. "We will own our jotería!" she belts out—almost singing—and the crowd whoops with delight and joy.

Jotería is a word that defies exact translation, a derogatory term reclaimed by queer Mexican and Latinx communities. Its closest corollary in English might be *faggotry*, crossed with *sissyness*, encompassing a range of gay, trans, and queer transgressions of the status quo. To own our jotería is to embrace what society has denigrated in us, to relish it, to see it as the power source it was always meant to be. We own our jotería—our transness, our euphoria, our queer AF genders, the erotic truths Lorde called an "assertion of the life force," the body-and-soul truths that have always been in us, as natural as breath—and in that owning we plug into a power source. We can draw on that power source for everything we do. Political work. Art-making. Love. Community-building. Family-making. Sex. Healing. Prayer, if we're moved to pray. The sheer pleasure of being fully present and real in the moment. And, of course, the great unending project of weaving a freer future for our people, one bright strand or step or word at a time.

//

At the TransLatin@ Coalition, Bamby and I finally settle down for our interview. We speak mostly in Spanish as she recounts her brutal childhood. Growing up in Guadalajara, Mexico, she endured poverty, sexual assault, transphobic violence, sex work, and police harassment from an early age. Later, after arriving in the US at sixteen, she would continue to face sexual violence, addiction, and incarceration in prisons and immigrant detention centers before becoming an activist and leader for trans and immigrant rights. Her story is wrenching, and immensely inspiring. She has been interviewed many times by now, including for the documentary *TransVisible: The Bamby Salcedo Story* and HBO's *The Trans List*. She is no stranger to questions about her past.

Still, when I ask her about gender euphoria in childhood, she pauses. She goes quiet for a moment, turning inward, as if searching for a way to respond. And then, she shares the story of the first time she ever wore a dress. She was twelve years old. She had already experienced, in her words, "a lot of things a child should not see." She found a group of queer and trans youth, ages twelve to eighteen, who gathered in the park. One night, this group decided to attend a party at a local gay rights organization. During the day, the organization provided HIV prevention and other resources, and by night they hosted community events.

"We went to somebody's place. I put a dress on. My first time. It was a long white dress, too. It was beautiful. At that moment, I felt as if I was Cinderella. It was just beautiful."

At this point, for the first and only time in the interview, Bamby weeps. For a while, she doesn't speak. I stay silent, holding space for her. The moment blossoms open; Bamby's face turns tender, transported back in time to that sanctuary of a party in Guadalajara, with the DJ and festive lights.

"I felt beautiful, ready to face the world. Like: I'm here. It was the best. That night was magical. It marked my life. Such moments mark you for life."

She looks deeply at me. I meet her gaze. We sit inside the memory together, bathed in afternoon light. Seeing each other. Seeing the white dress. Seeing what it could mean to be whole, to be fully alive.

AN INCOMPLETE HISTORY OF TRANS IMMORTALITY

ZEYN JOUKHADAR

Most of us don't have the luxury
of believing ourselves entitled to the future.

//

From the Great Above she opened her ear to the
Great Below.
From the Great Above the goddess opened her ear to
the Great Below.
From the Great Above Inanna opened her ear to the
Great Below . . .
Inanna abandoned heaven and earth to descend to
the underworld.

INANNA: QUEEN OF HEAVEN AND EARTH, TRANSLATED
BY DIANE WOLKSTEIN AND SAMUEL NOAH KRAMER

My future self sets the briefcase on the lunch table and clicks it
open, revealing two syringes of silver liquid. It's been eighteen,
maybe twenty years since this dream. Future Me has long auburn

hair, a terrible dye job I won't attempt until after college, in the bathroom sink of a ratty apartment. They pull a syringe from the briefcase, tap out the air, and say only: *A vaccination against what's to come.*

Most of us don't have the luxury of believing ourselves entitled to the future. Most of us—especially people of color living in a white supremacist society and world—are constrained to the past, if we are even allowed a past. The world is always ready to write of us in the past tense.

You might ask why I'm writing about trans immortality when, every day, every month, every year, more trans people are dying than ever. Let me put it to you this way. On July 9, 1975, thirty-three-year-old Dutch performance artist Bas Jan Ader set off from Cape Cod to cross the Atlantic in a thirteen-foot sailboat named the *Ocean Wave*. Nine months later, the unmanned vessel was found floating bow-down off the Irish coast. Ader was never found. His absence itself became the second part of his unfinished triptych *In Search of the Miraculous*. I suppose that if he hadn't risked death, even had he arrived to England, his arrival would not have been a miracle. Miracles are considered miracles only if terrible things would have happened in their absence. The cost is proportional to the miraculousness.

Terrible things happen all the time, I assure you, of which most of us know nothing. My question is what we do with unanswered prayers. Any history I tell of trans life, carrying that life into the future, will be incomplete because most of our histories are unknown, erased, or illegible to the cis arbiters of historical knowledge. No: I am not interested, here, in salvaging a recountable history. I want to know what happens to those of us whose names aren't treasured up in books or social media or candlelight vigils or other people's mouths, because most of us suffer without ever being immortalized. Like a mycelial network, we are connected by the thing that underlies us, but we may not realize it. One of us springs free of the earth in a field of potatoes; another parts the slipsoil of a mountainside, seeking siblings. We are ancient, though I'm not sure it matters. The oldest living organism is a lichen, a composite of an alga and a fungus, pulsing away undisturbed on a rock in Greenland for more than eight thousand years, growing only a centimeter in the course of a century.

A century!

We have the internet now, and all its fascists, and there are as many futures and pathways to them as you can possibly imagine. The future isn't linear; it's branching, various, multiplicitous as the lichen. What I want to know is what we do with a past, dense and painful and complicated, that refuses pat eulogy. I want to know how to hold the unknowable weight of trans suffering without erasing its hope. How many of my transcestors spent entire lifetimes bobbing along sweeping hearths, spreading duvet covers, slicing onions to feed a man and a child—lonesome and absorbed and convinced we were the only ones?

Future Me must have known about the basement rental, about the house centipedes and the boyfriend who kept a long knife in the bedside drawer. Future Me must have known about the bright, lonely apartment after that one, the man who hung crosses above all the doors. Maybe you've heard of the lesser-known Saint Agnes, the one from Rome, the patron saint of girls, chastity, virgins, gardeners, and victims of sexual abuse. When she refused the advances of her wealthy suitors, she was condemned to be dragged naked through the streets and raped in a brothel. Her hagiography claims she prayed as she was dragged, that her hair grew so long it covered her, that her would-be rapists were struck blind. Consider the cloak of her hair, the unburnt stake and pyre, the soldier unsheathing his sword. Consider the dozen or so men rubbing in terror at their eyes, the cries of darkness, their sudden night. And Saint Agnes standing there, thinking, *Now? Now you come?*

The Sumerian goddess Inanna, who descended into hell to offer her condolences to her sister Ereshkigal after the death of her husband, the Bull of Heaven, was said to have the power to change the gender of those who worshipped her, and people who might today be called transfeminine—the *galli*—performed rituals in her temples. In the Sumerian poem that describes her descent into the underworld, Inanna enters the throne room of her sister Ereshkigal, naked and bowed low. Inanna is not welcomed, but struck. Her body becomes meat, emptied. Her corpse is hung from a hook on the wall. For Inanna, time stops.

When my beard started growing in, I couldn't shake the feeling that I had been returned to my sixteen-year-old body. Like many trans people, I joked I'd become a vampire. My skin grew soft and acne-spotted; I rode my bike at night for miles and miles. The problem was not that I was thirty-three according to my birth certificate, but that sixteen was not a good age for me. There were things that happened to me at sixteen that I had worked very hard to forget, and apparently they lived in that pubertal body, the one I'd come back for at last. I washed my face twice a day, relived the desperate, lonely knot of driving past a high school boyfriend's house, the one everyone knew was gay before I did. This is the boyfriend who once wrote me into a story as a muscular, effeminate man flipping his dark hair in the wind. If I think too hard about the details of this story, it seems to wink out of existence, as though it is too incredible to have happened. We had a bad breakup. I thought love was a boulder and clung to people to convince myself that I existed. I needed the version of myself that existed in this boy's eyes. Without it, I feared I'd slide off the face of the earth. Which is very nearly what happened.

In a fable whose roots and versions span South and West Asia and parts of North Africa, a child is girled at birth, grows into an adolescent, and is betrothed to a man. The adolescent—still a child, really—prays to God to be changed into a boy.

Instead, a jinni answers. The jinni tells the child they may swap genders, so long as they swap back later. The child receives the jinni's penis and testicles, presumably what is meant by the word *sex*, and grows into a man. The man falls in love. The man is happy. He dreads the moment when he will have to swap back. But one day, the *jinniyah* returns. "I have broken the seal of the package with which I was entrusted," she says. She has become pregnant and cannot swap back.

As a child I did not think to want a penis. I understood my body as a thing to be redeemed, like sinners. Something in me had been opened by force, and I blamed this violation for God's great silence. *God*, I would pray outside my mother's church with my eyes shut tight, *God, come.* There was no rest of the prayer.

Bodies may be designed to live, but they aren't designed to last. Shortly after, at ten, I began to flood two and three overnight pads. I bled through the mattress. I missed school. I learned to swallow ibuprofen before it turned bitter. I learned the mercy of the body, that too much pain will make you pass out. I learned you can live in the land of pain, be hung from its rack and not die.

Scientists say endometriosis can be as painful as active labor, even a heart attack. I saw many, many doctors. A partial list of the doctors' suggestions: Motrin, Tylenol, squid ink, heating pads, meditation, antidepressants, anticonvulsants, birth control, prayer, valerian, chamomile, ginger, oxycodone, pregnancy. *One day*, I thought, *I will be dead. Then I will not be in pain.*

Awareness of death is an awareness of the future. Maybe your particular sick will not kill you. Still, other people design futures and fail to invite you.

Genetics, I learned during my doctoral studies, tells us that immortality is to ensure that one's offspring see the future—that is, unless you are a cancer cell, or a clump of endometrium on the run, clinging to bowel or bladder like a bank robber holed up in a roadside motel. I never had the right body to be a child. I didn't want to become someone else; I wanted a different history, which would have ensured a different future. As a chronically ill trans child and, now, a chronically ill trans adult who doesn't want to use my body to carry children, I will never be my parents' treasured immortality. I only know what it means to be the ghost of their want.

What do I do with the version of myself that remains suspended in pain? What do I do with the past selves who live in this body that slips through time? The more famous Saint Agnes, Chiara's sister, fled to her sister's convent to avoid a marriage. When the family came to yank her from the altar, her body became heavy as iron, and she was saved. In the fable of the jinn, the man is happy. He keeps his penis. It is a miracle.

In fairy tales and epics, two things lie beyond the realm of the human: the demonic and the divine. Stories of miraculous gender transformations occur in both fables and historical documents going back thousands of years. In a 2015 doctoral thesis entitled "(Trans)Culturally Transgendered: Reading Transgender Narratives in (Late) Imperial China," scholar Wenjuan Xie catalogs events of girled children transformed into boys or men because of their families' piety or sacrifice as far back as 487 BCE. Here, too, though, bodies like mine are objects, rather than subjects: Typically, the family wants a son in place of a daughter.

French trans artist and art historian Clovis Maillet writes in *Les Genres Fluides* about how medieval convents were havens for white transmasc and gender-nonconforming people assigned female at birth, though the same didn't work for transfems. To strive for the divine was to strive for maleness. In Europe in the Middle Ages, to be male was to be human, and therefore neutral; in a way, only women "had" gender as a modifying trait. In certain illustrations, women were labeled as a kind of animal. Because of the link between masculinity and virtue, the (white) body was sometimes deemed irrelevant. In what feels like a prelude to modern Western conceptions of the split between gender and the body, Saint Francis loses nothing of his manhood when Santa Chiara dreams of being breastfed by him. Italian art historian Chiara Frugoni recounts the story: "The saint drew out from his breast a teat and said to the virgin Chiara: 'Come, receive and suck.' And sucking it, that which flowed from it was so sweet and delectable, that she could in no way explain it . . . and taking in her hands that which remained in her mouth, it [the milk] seemed to her gold so clear and shining that all was seen in it, almost as in a mirror" (translation mine).

The list of trans saints is already long and well documented. And though other people's eyes are not a prerequisite for existence, there is something profound about being looked into like Francis's golden milk. Chaza Cherafeddine, in *Divine Comedy* (2010), photographed Beiruti trans women and cast them as the fantastical Buraq, the winged, human-faced steed of the Prophet, peace be upon him, dazzling in emerald and ruby feathers. That said, on the ceiling of the dome of the cupola of the Cathedral of Florence, Vasari's and Zuccari's angels of *The Last Judgment* are white twinks with flat chests and smooth cheeks, while their demons are brown, purple, green, hairy as goats. Their bodies are adorned with breasts and penises, their fire-tipped spears plunged into the nether regions of tortured souls. In this version of the universe, my friends and I are having the world's most epic orgy in hell.

I won't romanticize the survival of my transcestors. Had I been born a century earlier, a centimeter in the history of lichen, I might not have survived. In this version of my life, I am declared possessed by male jinn, seized by malevolent spirits. In this version of my life, I write out passages from the Qur'an, submerge them in water, and drink the dissolved ink. In this version of my life, I pray.

The Catholic Church believes in the concept of a victim soul, those chosen by God to suffer for the redemption of humankind. This isn't something the church declares; the person alone knows. Santa Gemma Galgani of Lucca was the daughter of a Tuscan pharmacist, orphaned at eighteen after her father, mother, and brother all died of tuberculosis. The disease would take her, too, at twenty-five. She is the patron saint of pharmacists, parachutists, orphans, those with back pain and migraines.

She was said to levitate and received the stigmata at twenty-one, a precocious, teacher's-pet saint.

A victim soul.

Everyone knows how to be happy but you, I scolded myself for much of my twenties, because I believed happiness to be an act of will. The only video that exists of me dancing was made at a residency on Ohlone land, to a recording of Umm Kulthum singing. Minutes before, an Argentinian artist had taken a pair of scissors and cut into my white T-shirt while I moved, turning my sleeves into curtains of knots, creating a keyhole across my sternum and a slash on each flank. I didn't ask him to do this, so he can't know I want to excuse myself from my life. In the video, you can't tell. I'm not a good dancer, but in this video, I look like a girl who knows how to dance. I wanted to make a copy of myself that could live without me in it. I don't appear in the eye of the camera. I am buried beneath it like a seed.

Little more than a year after the video, out as trans to my close friends and partner but still trying to convince myself I can live with my dysphoria, I'm walking through the city of Lucca after a couple of glasses of wine, having forgotten all about Santa Gemma. It is two days before Christmas. Though I won't unravel my feelings about hormones for another two years, I keep telling myself I will find a way through my exhaustion and dissociation. I try to convince myself that I could even give birth, though it's unclear whether my body is capable of pregnancy and I don't want to find out. Doctors tell me testosterone will destroy my fertility, though this isn't true, and I've just found out it's illegal for same-sex couples to adopt in my partner's country, Italy. Maybe I could go away in my head, I reason, smile at strangers. I'd shut my testosterone canisters in a cabinet. I'd stay very still. I conjure a hypothetical life in which I have a partner so grateful for babies that they look at me every day and smile. They smile so hard they cry, smile so hard they have to go to special doctors because their face begins to hurt from smiling. I know you can survive your body being taken from you. People have been looking through me like a window all my life. *Courage, hold your breath. Glaze over like a lake in winter. You won't feel a thing.*

The wine dulls the cold, but still we turn into a narrow street, out of the wind. A portrait hangs over the lintel of a door. I recognize Gemma's upturned gaze, her black frock and folded hands. I sit down on the steps of the house opposite and command myself to cry. I cannot. I berate myself for being tipsy and unhealed. In this house, a saint's hands and feet began to bleed. God passed through Gemma and transformed her. I'm still waiting to be touched.

After the meat of Inanna's body is hung on the rack, Ninshubur, her handmaiden, dresses herself as a beggar. She tears at her eyes, her mouth, her thighs. She sets out for Nippur and petitions Enlil at his temple, who denies her. She goes to Ur, to the temple of Nanna, who turns her away.

Finally, in Eridu, Enki grieves for her plea. Father Enki picks bits of soil from under his fingernails and transforms them into a *kurgarra* and a *galatur*, beings "neither male nor female." Giving them the food and water of life, he tells them, "Go to the underworld. Enter the doors like flies."

The next time Future Me came, I dreamed of him in a nightclub. I wore a sparkly purple mini dress I'd recently given away to another trans friend and my three-and-a-half-inch black plastic heels with the cork platforms. He looked dangerous and sleek, and I cursed him. *God*, I thought, *I am going to be beautiful*, then bolted, terrified, through the crowd. If I stared too long he might leap down my throat, sprout black hair on my thighs, swell the muscle in my shoulders, unfurl the veins in the backs of my hands. An ecstatic fire would enter me, a joy I could not permit myself under any circumstances. The pain would kill me, I feared, were I able to feel anything else.

Santa Lucia is the patron saint of the blind, but also of a long list of others: martyrs, saddlers, stained glass workers, the town of Perugia, even (God help us) authors. In the northern Italian town where I now live with my partner, Santa Lucia's feast day used to be a bigger celebration than Christmas. Something real still remains of her, or at least it used to, when the saint used to roam the streets of little Bergamasco towns in a long dress and veil of white lace. Everyone knew the one who came to the elementary school was fake, my partner tells me, like a shopping-mall Santa. But the one who floated through the town couldn't be written off. The children would tell her the gifts they wanted as she passed, and Lucia, silent, would incline her head. Several women took turns wearing her white dress. The body was a door for the sacred. Lucia's veil made a woman into something else.

According to legend, Lucia was a Sicilian woman from Syracuse who was martyred when Diocletian gouged out her eyes in the third century. Her feast day was originally celebrated on the winter solstice, her blindness symbolizing the darkness of the longest night of the year into which she—the name *Lucia* itself derived from the Latin *lux*—bore the light. Only in the fifteenth century does she begin to appear eyeless, bearing two lidless orbs on a plate. Francesco del Cossa depicts her lifting a delicate stem from which another set of eyes blossom, like lilies.

The light would have been different in the years my partner saw Santa Lucia. The streetlamps were all sodium vapor then, yellow-orange, not the penetrating blue-white of LEDs. When I left home for college, the only blue lights were the emergency call buttons scattered around campus. There was one trail where there was no blue light, a trail leading between certain campus buildings and certain dorms through a small wood. The boys called this the "rape trail."

Most cities have LED streetlamps now, and the night doesn't look the same. The light has changed, disappearing the shadows I remember. Yet I still fear the trees.

I meet Future Me again at a barbecue. In this dream, he has his arm around my partner and a cup in his hand. He is laughing. He has denser stubble, a more angular jaw. I am jealous of him because he is happier, more charming, more beautiful than me. I am jealous of him because he lives in a beautiful future into which I cannot follow.

He comes to me in my midthirties, as governments around the world are doing everything in their power to eliminate trans life and parenthood via sterilization requirements, abortion bans, smearing us as pedophiles, making it illegal for queer and trans people to adopt, listing us incorrectly on our children's birth certificates (and our own documents), and criminalizing life-saving health care for both trans children and, increasingly, adults. He comes to me as right-wing politicians attempt to outlaw the imagining of trans futures.

Future Me is slowly replacing Present Me. I'm not saying I

was ever another person. I'm saying some part of me, the pilot-light version of myself, kept me alive when living was too painful to do. For years I assumed everything that happened during those dissociated decades was lost, mercifully. But once I began testosterone, memory surged up from deep freeze. I once tried to reenvision my childhood traumas with my present body, and for a few seconds I closed the distance on my past self with vicious clarity: There I was, the boy and his pain, and finally, terrifyingly, I understood myself to be human. But the feeling was slippery; it fell away at once, and I lost it again. To dissociate is to become a mirror, the surface of a windless lake. Who, exactly, had been raped? Was a younger me still trapped there, waiting for a miracle?

Time is a spiral with its layers pressed together. Ibn 'Arabi describes time as an eternal circle. All points on the circle, though distinct, remain in touch with eternity. The past is not separate from the future, but part of it. If the past slips into my present, I see no reason why the future shouldn't slip back to visit me. Only the future is slippery, too. A transition, like a novel, is a risk. The real dislodges the fantasy, destroys it, debases it by existing. But the real is tangible, at least. You can work with the real. A transition, unlike the fact of being trans, requires you to choose yourself. I would learn only later that it also requires you to relinquish your fantasies not only of who you will become, but of who you've been.

My transition will never be finished. I am not following a line from one binary gender to another, but moving laterally, diagonally, inwardly, spiraling through time in my ever-changing, ever-returning body. Even melancholy, in this skin, is sweet. The boy I exiled comes alive in my face. I am eroding a fantasy of who

I thought I was, crumbling it like wet sand, revealing the boy banished to the self behind the self. The boy who kept very still, frozen, so we might one day live.

If what Ibn ʿArabi says is true, then I possess immortality—like eternity—in this very moment, in my very body. Listen: I am trying to arrive at the miracle by the door of my trans flesh. I will not believe them when they write that I am dead.

The kurgarra and the galatur find the queen of the underworld naked and in labor, moaning, her hair "swirled around her head like leeks." When she groans, "Oh! Oh! My belly!" they groan, "Oh! Oh! Your belly!" She cries, "My back!" They cry, "Your back! Your heart! Your liver!"

Bewildered, she asks who they are to share in her pain, offering them the river and the fields as a reward. But they ask only for the corpse hung on the wall, and the reward is granted.

The kurgarra sprinkles the food of life on the corpse.

The galatur sprinkles the water of life on the corpse.

Inanna rises.

If immortality is a possibility that exists from moment to moment, perhaps practicable immortality is a hope in the future as a reachable place. Once I writhed in bed, wondering if the pain—like the future—was all in my head. I clasped my belly and stared at my father's paintings. I, too, wanted to be an artist. I didn't have the word *trans* then, but I was convinced I would die young. I believed the only way not to disappear was to make art, as though by making something beautiful I could locate God. Bas Jan Ader set off from Cape Cod in a thirteen-foot sailboat and was never seen again. Maybe the beautiful future, like eternity, is an asymptote we approach only once we accept that we may never reach it.

My partner, Italian visual artist Matteo Rubbi, once made a work called *Il Muro*, "the wall": A single person supports a wooden wall that would otherwise fall, holding it upright with the force of their outstretched arms. I can't pluck my past selves from the rack of pain, just as I will never know most of the trans siblings who were afforded no miracles. I came back for myself, as we come for one another. The self who haunts me teaches me that our beautiful futures will not abandon us so long as we hold them aloft, like my partner's impossible wall, with our hands.

This, at least, is what I tell myself, and plant my feet.

IN MY WORST NIGHTMARES, MY FATHER TRANSITIONS

KAIA BALL

She apologizes for all the vitriol she ever flung at me,
crying thick tears through false eyelashes.

I. Father

In my worst nightmares, my father transitions.

In life, we are many years estranged, per his wishes. He has made his feelings on my "gender deviance" clear. The fiery drama of the fallout of our nuclear family has long since cooled to ash, long-ago shouting matches stretched into years of silence.

And yet.

In these dreams, her beauty is effortless. She moves with supreme Black elegance, each gesture power incarnate. The perfect shade of foundation blends the sun-scarred skin of her forehead into her cheeks. A hairline I once watched recede is handily buried beneath luscious curls, voluminous as mine were before I hacked them off. Even her five-o'clock shadow has been put to rest.

She kneels before me, her shimmering skirt unwrinkled by the movement. She holds my hands with nails lacquered violet.

My father always loved violet.

She apologizes for all the vitriol she ever flung at me, crying thick tears through false eyelashes. Gentle and contrite, she apologizes for calling me a cross-dresser, a dyke, a homosexual, a gender bender, a transvestite. Through lips painted by artists, she begs for my forgiveness, admitting in the same breath that she could never earn it.

Her humility is palpable, as is her beauty. Her regret is tangible, as is her grace. I stand, stone-faced, and grant her no reprieve.

In my worst nightmares, my father transitions. There, she is a better person than me.

And she's better at being trans than I am.

II. Elder

My mother once told me, "You are your true self when you're on a date with a boy. When you go too long without putting on makeup, it's like you lose sight of who you really are."

I sometimes wondered if my mother would've been happier with a mirror for a daughter. I know for a fact she would've been happier with a daughter, but we get what we get, and she got me.

I only rarely saw my mother without a full face of makeup, and never in the full force of natural daylight. She had the art form down pat, just a few moments needed before sunrise to put her face on. Bright lips, thin brows, plump lashes, foundation in the lightest shade on the market. She wanted the same for me, claiming that it was part of a woman's hygiene. I refused, hence her insistence that I had lost sight of my true self.

To this day, I've never seen her natural hair color. She started dyeing it in high school. If photos existed of her any younger, I can't recall them. Maybe I was never shown them. Her hair is the exact same shade of box blond in her wedding photos as on the day of my disowning more than two decades later.

She spends my childhood bemused by my mixed hair, constantly trying to tame it, straighten it, relax it, beat it into submission. Dye it to look like hers. She wrecks my curls, over and over, until I am big enough to hide, to force her to pick a different battle.

My father tells me I should be grateful. Girls are lucky, he says, that they get to wear makeup at all. He revels in the few opportunities he has to be onstage, eyeliner accentuating bright green eyes, blush high on his cheekbones.

We might show up late to church, but we look good when we get there. I am the eldest child of the lot of us, an octopus wrangling clip-on ties to shirt necks that refused to starch. The memories, resistant to chronology, swell and shrink. There's four of us, then seven, then six. A slew of mixed kids, our hair brown and black and ginger, tan and pale and freckled, bookended by a pale black man in violet and a far paler white woman with box-blond hair.

After the sacrament, administered by teenage boys in ill-fitting black jackets, the congregation splits by gender, then by age. Gender lies at the center of Mormonism, so say our scriptures.

In the '90s, church leaders said so explicitly in a document titled *The Family: A Proclamation to the World*: "Gender is an essential characteristic of individual pre-mortal, mortal, and eternal identity and purpose." Mormons the world over were to take that as eternally pertinent scripture like any line of the Bible. Eve supped on forbidden fruit, David kissed Jonathan, gender is who you are and why you exist.

Gender shone in every aspect of Mormon life. At church my brothers learned to rake, grill, hike, change tires, build fires, wield the mystical powers of the priesthood to heal the sick and raise a family.

My sisters and I learned to sew, knit, crochet, cook. I cleaned the building, gathering up the Nerf darts left behind from the boys' playtimes. I minded children smaller than the child I was, mended skinned knees and scraped elbows. I wore dresses, skirts, and kept my hair long enough to cover my shoulders and collarbone.

A sincere devotee, I was prepared for the life ahead of me. Once a Mormon boy decided that I was a good enough match to raise a family with, I would bear his children. After death, his righteousness would earn him a planet, and I would fill it to the brim with offspring. Rumors swirled at summer camp that if a very kind husband found you, he might let you help pick out the planet's name.

I hoped that our planet would be named something nice and that my husband would be even nicer. Whenever I imagined him, he shone as a silhouette of blinding light, intangible and scalding.

That document was likely named *The Family* because it tackled another subject heavy on the minds and hearts of Mormons at the turn of the millennium. It opened with the line, "We, The Church of Jesus Christ of Latter-day Saints, solemnly proclaim that marriage between a man and a woman is ordained of God."

III. Cover

I nightmare of three subjects: My father, Black and celestial. My mother, white and earthen. And the day following the day I got outed. My parents managed to corner and confront me during that brief visit home from college, a two-pronged attack.

The shocking revelation of my dykehood was an open secret only a Mormon's mouth can hold. I watched in grotesque fascination as it bumped against my parents' lips, carrot-raisin-lime-gelatin sloshing in their cheeks.

I wound up, during this lecture turned terror, holding my youngest sibling, feeding them bottled formula. They were an infant I had met a couple days previously. I was a college sophomore. The many siblings between us were hidden somewhere. Perhaps they lurked in the depths of the house, invisible witnesses to the lurid affair. Perhaps they were at school, oblivious to the whole thing.

I hold this child, a stranger, for the entirety of this memory, this nightmare, this horrifically mundane Armageddon. Their weight pins me to a rickety rocking chair as the hours stretch on. Their sleepy peace keeps my voice small, my body still as I cradle them.

"Of all the childish choices," says my father. He loves science fiction and fantasy. He probably would've loved the book I'm writing now, six years later. It has dragons, and wizards, and pigeons.

"You're too young to know," says my mother. She was married at twenty-one. She had me at twenty-two. She used to teach puppetry classes. She likes to sew costumes, astronauts and explorers and dragons. We all really like dragons.

"You're rushing into this," sighed my father.

"Being gay?" I whispered.

"You're being so dramatic," scolded my mother.

From their first date to their engagement, my parents courted for six weeks.

They were both enrolled in a theater program at a Mormon university, perfectly ensconced in a cocoon of faith and art. My father would proudly show off a photograph of the single night he spent in drag, some thirty years ago now. "I should've shaved my legs," he'd always say. "I looked so wonderful. That hair, the lipstick, the fishnets. But I wish I'd shaved my legs!"

They met reading across each other for parts in a Shakespeare play, a moment so magical they could never remember the name of the play or the parts they read. Just their chemistry: They connected so resonantly that when they found themselves knee-deep in a passionate argument on a stranger's balcony months later, they knew their love was meant to be.

"You've always hated men," says my father. He cites my middle school bullying, shoving boys half my size aside, wrenching their long hair to their knees.

"You're taking the easy way out," declared my mother. "Sure. Every girl wants to cut all her hair off and raise kids with her best friend. But growing up means making the responsible choice."

In my teenage years, my mother expressed concerns over my having so many sapphic friends. She told me that they would need to make their choice soon, lest the rest of their life be doomed. "No one gets to stay a child forever. Growing up means choosing to be responsible. Choosing to love men. It's what I did, just like everyone else."

Slowly, over two and a half hours, the shape of it takes root.

My parents are furious that I am refusing to make the difficult decision to eschew the temptations of homosexuality in favor of a righteous life of devotion to Mormon Jesus. They made their choice long ago in one another and have been donning masculinity and femininity and heteronormativity ever since. You, they point accusatory fingers at me, need to do the same.

Over the next couple of tumultuous years, we will fight and scream and cry and bicker as my hair gets lopped off and my dresses become hand-me-downs and my earrings are converted into cufflinks. My father will rage when he sees unisex dress socks on a Christmas list, screaming that I'm not a man and I'll never be one. My mother will cry when I tell her I won't wear the glittery plaids she got me as a replacement for the thrifted flannels that swallowed my wardrobe in early college.

When I am inevitably, uproariously, explosively disowned, it is followed by the total silence of people who have said all they needed to say.

IV. Other

A molecular biologist, I dutifully spend a chunk of the pandemic in laboratories, hunched over benches, scrubbing the body raw. Afterward I bounce from gig to gig. Retail. Childcare. Freelance copywriting. Substitute teaching.

My friends, my loved ones ask if I'm sure, if it's worth the risk. I'm an obnoxiously effusive type, so social jobs suit me well. But the last time I worked retail, the public did me the dubious honor of teaching me the lesson that it's dangerous to look like me, to have my voice, and most of all to use it.

"They're just kids," I remind my friends. There's nothing a thirteen-year-old can do to hurt me worse than the grown man who dropped a fridge on me when he heard my butch body speak in soprano.

That dissonance visibly resonates in my reflection as I array myself carefully, the attention of a bomb defuser trained on an outfit assembled from Walmart clearance and Ross.

Shoes too long in the toe and too stubby in the ball have been my companion for seven moves, going on eight next month. I tug on a thrifted polo, scratchy despite the softener I've thrown at it.

I've done my best to take in the khakis, but the stitches are visible in places that make the amateur alterations uncomfortably obvious. The hems are both uneven and far too high, showing off, depending on the day, several inches of novelty Pikachu socks or my unshaved calves. The good dress socks are in the wash, of course. I also somehow misaligned the sewing on the seat of this pair of pants, so it's somehow both too baggy and yet too tight on the crack. Meant for a different set of equipment, not meant for my curves, not meant to hold me.

Once upon a time, when my body stretched and swelled, my mother sewed clothes to flatter it. She made me dresses and blouses that fit. My brothers wore hand-tailored vests, my father's pants mended and hemmed.

She messaged me on LinkedIn for my birthday this past year, one of the few digital places I had overlooked in the four years since our estrangement. The message sat unopened, but I looked at the sewing machine, the too-short pants with uneven hems. Wondered about a family in perfectly tailored clothes, perfectly flattering their bodies.

I wondered what my mother would look like in a suit.

That hair that was the subject of so many fights with my parents has been dyed to hell now, curls murdered by bleach and only now gasping back to life. The sunshine yellow of the summer is resistant to resurrection, but I'm trying to keep it up till the holidays. The kids love the yellow, especially the little ones, and it's been a long season for them.

Now low on time and rushing, I pin my custom name tag on. It only lists a little over the Lycra of my exhausted sports bra.

Mx. Ball
They/Them

No, the kids were nothing to be afraid of.

The adults, on the other hand . . .

When the local high school principal called me, he spoke carefully, each word measured. I tried to match his pace, unsure of my footing. A rookie substitute teacher in a large district could hardly feel that this call was a good omen.

A parent had contacted him and the school multiple times in the past day to complain about . . . the man hesitates.

Each of the following syllables rolls off his tongue like boulders. "It's my understanding that you use they and them pronouns?"

My stomach drops. *Ah. This again.*

That awkward, and ultimately pointless, phone call with the principal was the second incident in the past six months. A different superior, a different job, a different parent, complaining about my existence being "age inappropriate." "Gender," says the last boss, "is just something we don't talk about here."

"I'm not bringing it up." I desperately want to make eye contact with her. I can't look up from my shoes. "The kids keep asking."

The ghost of my mother, reaming out a superintendent, hovers over my right shoulder, ranting about school bus safety. Someone's getting fired tomorrow.

A manager rolls his eyes at me when I correct him, sotto voce. He tells me that it's not grammatically correct to be multiple people.

The ghost of my father stands thunderously before me. Dictionaries are splayed next to him, Webster wielded like a rapier.

My parents were educators. Probably still are. That's a quirk of estrangement: People wind up caught in amber the moment of relationship terminus.

I've attended their classes, their lectures, their sermons. Watched them gather up a disparate audience and palm them, turn a room on the pad of their finger. *Laugh*, commands my father, and the room erupts. *Weep*, sniffles my mother, and the crowd is somber.

They'd be better at this, nags the flash of myself warped in car windows, the glimmer of a person in the cheap plastic of a child's sunglasses.

They'd stand up for themselves, I sigh as another diversity and inclusion coordinator calls me an upstanding young woman.

They'd have something to say, something quick and bright and real.

They'd sew perfect clothes, strike perfect poses, speak in perfect voices.

They'd be better at this, as men or women or whatever oddity I am.

They'd overtake me in an instant.

V. Mother

Dreams of my mother find us walking on the rocky beach of her parents' old home. They moved out of that wooden house years ago, but when I think of my grandparents I still remember their tiny chunk of bay on the west end of Puget Sound.

Baby girl of six brothers, my mother is dressed in obvious hand-me-downs. A canvas jacket sits heavy on her collarbone, a thick flannel poking out past her hips. She moves with surety in thick galoshes across the uneven beach. Her hair is tucked under a handmade beanie, Seahawks green and blue. She smells like grit and sulfur, a slight tint of shrimpy wet coming in from the west.

On our trek, I stuff my pockets with every chunk of beach that glimmers. Quickly I am bowlegged from the weight of them, and look to my mother for her help in carrying my quickly expounding bounty of treasures. "Mom—"

"Shh." Her attention is trained on the mouth of the bay. Her cheeks are pockmarked. She has crow's feet. She wears no mascara, no lipstick. She's wearing glasses.

I'm smug with her. "I thought you had 20/20." I've needed mine since I was six. She lorded her perfect vision over me.

She rolls her eyes, pointing with one hand, the other reaching for a holster on her belt. "I needed to watch the whale."

It was a legend in our home. Once, when my mother was a teen, a juvenile whale got wedged in the tiny bay in my grandparents' backyard. It fell to them and the neighbors to keep her calm, keep her wet, and holler at the idiot Coast Guard for trying to bring their massive honking ships into tiny inlets they wouldn't be able to maneuver out of.

Now I can see it, too, the whale trapped in a deceptively inviting inlet at the north end of the bay. She thrashes, weeps, splashing and screaming and crying.

My mother moves down the beach in a way I didn't know her legs moved, the way Paul Bunyan ate up the country, the way a railroad moves a family from New York to Missouri, the way a road trip brings you home. She wades into the water, taller than an evergreen, as mighty as her lumberjack father, arms wide for the trapped beast. Gentle, she calms the whale, rubbing at the sore areas where craggy rock has torn at marine hide.

My mother takes a few steps back, stance firm, galoshes steady. At her belt materializes a rope, spun from pine needles and spidersilk, the corners of my grandparents' basement. With a heaving motion, the whale is wrangled, the rope thrown over my mother's shoulder.

Knees bent, head down, body set, my mother begins to heave. Step by Herculean step, the whale is pulled through the shallow bay according to her will, by the power of her determination. Her cheeks flush red from the effort. Her temples bulge. She snorts and grunts and sweats.

Halfway through her journey, a jostle of the rope whips her beanie off. For the first time in my life, I see my mother's natural hair color.

It's the same as mine.

VI. Further

My suit, a deep emerald, slips on perfectly. A discerning eye can tell that it was tailored by someone minding my curves, squaring my shoulders, tapering to my calves. Silky florals flare in the lining of the jacket, more color than most men would ever dare.

It brings out the green in my eyes, an echo of my father's own. The parchment button-up sits on my hips just like the blouses my mother once sewed for me. When I take up the arm of my lover that night, my gold bangles will clang against their own jewelry, matching gold embroidery on their dress. We will dazzle, and network, and delight. We'll fling coded words past oblivious ears, knowing that even now we and our people live on the fringes of visibility, able to speak to one another privately in a crowded room.

If eyes narrow, if offered handshakes are rebuffed, if shoulders get bumped, I ignore them. It's a talent of mine, well practiced and often called upon. I perfected it on walks late at night, at long shifts behind the register, in line at the bank, at countless tribunals of the public eye. *Go on,* my smile dares them. *Give me, dyed hair and soft chest and high voice and all, a chance to be the bigger man.*

The children are starting to recognize me, towering above their teachers, booming voice and bright colors undeniable. I made a new friend down in Denver, and he says he'll coach me on hemming sometime in the new year. In the meantime I got new socks, boisterous and colorful. I affix my name tag, speak my name clearly. Half the time now the children have already alerted one another long before I get there—

"Oh, oh, it's *mix ball* today."

Little ones quietly pass me scraps of paper, pronouns scrawled in mechanical pencil. A young man pulls me aside to ask about binders, and hormones, and how I got so tall. Secret names are whispered to me, treasures received with the greatest of reverence.

I still, on occasion, catch glimpses of a diaphanous femme father in the sweet turn of my lips. Hints of a butch mother can still be found between my set shoulders, shifting to bear heavy burdens. But a simple examination of the wearing of the tread of my work boots serves as refutation to years of maladaptive fantasy. Those people never existed, and I am here, putting one sore foot in front of the other.

In my worst nightmares, my father transitions.

In my wildest dreams, my father transitions.

When I awaken, my father is but a man.

In a kinder world, my mother and my father have different titles, or the same ones. They got to be mother-fathers and father-mothers. They got to wear dresses and suits and makeup and neckties. They got to experiment with their genders in college and realized that they were happy as they were. They got to experiment in college and realized that the roles that they had been taught could never contain the magnitude of human spirit spilling out of them.

In a kinder world I am coached through a life beyond a binary by two people who never fit in one to begin with.

In this world, those of us who chose to sow transformation reap trans joy.

In this world, I am what they never had the strength, or love, or balls to be.

FUTURES

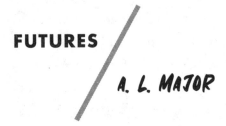

A. L. MAJOR

When I was a child, the future was a survival tool.

When I was a child, the future was a survival tool. I was a tender little one, goofy, gentle, not unlike I am now, but I was beaten quite severely for things I don't believe a child should be punished for, let alone harmed.

As an adult, I am acutely aware of the abuse I suffered as a child—that there are only a few spots on my body that haven't felt someone's rage, the force of a palm or the stinging kiss of a silver belt—and how devastating it is that even my face is no stranger to brutality, that on two separate occasions I can recall: a hand cocked back, delivering a blow that still reverberates through me like a long wail that only I can hear.

(Yet this isn't an essay about my trauma, I don't think.)

//

When I was a child, the future was a survival tool. Whenever I had trouble falling asleep on the twin mattress that I shared with my sister, I imagined the mansion I would one day own, its king-size bed, and its verdant garden, and the leggy palm trees that overlooked my large tennis court, where my husband—olive skin, green eyes, so classically handsome he doesn't need a personality—would play tennis in the mornings. My husband and I had three kids—one boy, one girl, one surprise, all wavy brown hair and brilliant white teeth.

This remarkably anodyne fantasy lulled me to sleep quite easily. In the morning, I would wake with little memory of that family or our time together, just the cloying sweetness of something that I might one day taste. Then with my eyes still blurry from such deep slumber, I would be forced to be a child again, bow-legged and ashy-kneed. Everyone told me I was a girl, but I never acted like one. I was stocky. I ran through new school shoes every few months—one semester even, tiring of how often I needed new shoes, my mother refused to buy me a new pair, and I was forced to walk around for several weeks with shoes that looked like open, hanging, desperate mouths; everywhere I went, those broken shoes made this awful *clack clack clack* sound, their broken jaws just *clack clack clack*ing against my feet. My friends would snicker, my teachers would snicker—their laughter is another shame that has built a home in me.

I also developed breasts before many of my peers; I tried to hide them by hunching my shoulders and wearing baggy dresses. Tactics, I suppose, I still use now. My mother employed a different tactic. One afternoon, she dragged me to the mall and forced me to try on training bras. While my mother chatted with the sales-person about my developing breasts, the awkward perky shape of them, and how expensive it was to raise children in this economy, these two strangers gossiping like old friends, I struggled with this ugly white strappy thing suffocating my chest. I knew something was changing, that I would be treated differently from then on, but I couldn't have known that I would grieve this change long after we left the mall and longer still after we returned home to that yellow house with the orange carpet and the bars on all of its windows.

I hated those bras, mostly because no one else my age wore them and so adults—my teachers, my mother's friends—would comment on the straps that would peek out from the neckline of my school dress. These weren't sexually inappropriate comments, at least not that I recall, more like shock or confusion that at such a young age—I was only eight or nine—my body was already unruly, unknowable, a dark earthy forest that needed to be tamed, burned if need be, and cultivated into the exact opposite of what it wanted to be. These adults and their comments incited such a burning revulsion (for the instruments that would be used to contain me) that without my mother knowing, every day I would pull down the bra's straps in a bathroom stall before morning class and wear the bra like a rubber band around my stomach through-out the school day. (And then everything was freedom, not yet the heavy weight of adulthood, just the body in motion, its sweat, the softness of my bare skin against light polyester fabric.)

During recess, I would con my friends into playing the paper game MASH just so I could cheat the outcomes I wanted. Other days, I would do palm-reading sessions, where I asserted psychic authority over the ridges and etchings of my friends' palms—how long they would live, how successful they would be in their careers, whether they would get married 'til death do them part.

My own palms tell two radically different futures. In one future, I live a long life; I achieve great career success, but my love life is in shambles. In the other, I am not quite as successful in my career. I have a love that sustains me, and my life line weakens about three-quarters of its way down my palm. I don't know if this means I will die young or if I will always be a little hidden from the world, just a faint scratch on the earth's palm and nothing more. But either way, at the end of the school day, I would pull the bra back up again over my breasts, wince at the restriction masquerading as support, and my mother—well, she never knew of any of this.

//

On difficult nights nowadays, I pop a melatonin and watch YouTube videos until I fall asleep—vlogs by people who live in their cars, unedited gameplay footage of 4X strategy games. Lately, I've become obsessed with collecting antique postcards, and so occasionally I watch videos of deltiologists sharing the collections that took their entire lives to acquire—and my dreams are always of a quiet nature, nothing I need to recall the next morning.

I used to love morning runs. Those were the days I felt most certain of my aliveness. When I lived in Massachusetts, I lived a five-minute walk from the Charles River path, which offered everything I needed for a run: length (the path is more than twenty miles long), flatness (mostly), trees (American elm, black oak, sugar maple), privacy (I hate running near high-traffic streets; I don't like strangers to see me struggle). I've never been a particularly fast runner, nor has running fast ever been my goal. I run to prove that my body is so much more capable than I believe it to be. A metaphor for life, I'm sure, a cliché even: how I begin every run exasperatedly, every inhale an assault, every second feeling like an hour, and though every part of me wants to stop, I push through until the pain is no longer unbearable, in fact is gone, and I feel the closest to free I'll ever feel.

(The body in motion. Its sweat. The softness of my bare skin against light cotton fabric.)

These mornings, I do not run. I lie in bed and refuse to drink water and I scroll through my social media feeds and I learn about famines and genocides and bans on trans healthcare and my body gets heavier until it's an anchor to the ocean of my grief and I lose those precious early hours, I miss out on those blissful runs, and the day is just one task after the other, after the other, until I put myself to sleep again.

//

The things I was certain I wanted as a child, I no longer desire in the same way, if at all. The huge mansion seems cold to me now—selfish, unnecessary. Those brilliant children, I don't know whether I have the patience to raise all three of them anymore, and most certainly I don't have the wealth. And that husband? I have left him in my old childhood bedroom, where the *Goosebumps* books and Disney VHS tapes live. This isn't uncommon—who in our generation has not had their childhood imagination kidnapped by *Saved by the Bell* and *Dawson's Creek*—but it surprises me, nevertheless, how different that childhood vision is from what my life turned out to be.

How many futures have I imagined for myself, and how many have I lost? How many more will I lose in this lifelong pursuit of growth and self-discovery?

I came out twice in my twenties. Once as queer and the second time as trans and nonbinary. Coming out as queer was easy. It was 2010. I was attending a former all-women's college in upstate New York. I played rugby—loosehead prop, tighthead prop, second row. I was a vegetarian. I loved (and love) Tracy Chapman and Ani DiFranco unironically—yes, I still love young Ani, even though old Ani tried to do that concert that one time on that slave plantation; there are some white folks I just don't know how to say goodbye to. All this to say that in the fall of 2010, the only person my queerness was a surprise to was me.

Coming out as trans was a different shock, more electrifying only because I was even less prepared for it. I had always been overconfident—self-assured to a fault. To discover that I didn't know myself, that perhaps I would never fully know myself, was profoundly humbling—and, at times, tiring. That year of figuring out my gender was such a sudden and urgent excavation. I was slowly approaching my late twenties. I was married and living in Massachusetts. I would go to work at a children's science museum, do a marketing job I never imagined for myself, and during my lunch breaks I would cry in the bathroom—for how lonely I felt those days, so very lonely as my marriage fell apart. I mourned so often, so privately and publicly, in this one bathroom, that I can still recall the colors of its tiles, how they were the deep, rich shades of a familiar forest that I have only ever visited in my dreams.

In between emails and team meetings where I strategized how to sell engineering curriculum to middle schools, I would retreat inward, crawl into my mind's tunnels and dig through every memory, pick over the fossils of my desires to see if I could discover that one missing bone, so sharp, so clean, that it could finally put me back together as whole.

(I fear I don't know what it means to be whole; if being whole is in itself an impossible future. I have shifted my needs to try and heal the wounds of so many people, I do not know what is mine anymore.

Am I too much for one partner? Or too little? Would I enjoy giving birth to a child if it didn't mean a losing—of body, of self? Could I love being pregnant, if I could also grieve the havoc such a miracle would wreak upon my body? And is that okay? To need things? To feel?

The future is as mutable as my answers to these questions. Some days, I know the answers with such startling clarity that I want to drop everything I'm doing and start making the future happen, stop overindulging and overspending, stop obsessing over people and things that do not serve me.

Most days, though, I am lazy, and every answer is simply a theory, and every theory is valid, completely plausible and yet never truly provable.)

//

I have struggled with debilitating anxiety all my life, and I think perhaps that has caused me to become overly dependent on the future. I've felt for a long time now that I'm in a holding pattern, waiting for the circumstances of my present to be better before I start doing anything about my future. I hate this about myself—that now my future has become a repository for all the desires that I deny myself in the present.

In the future, I will publish my novel.

In the future, I will run a marathon.

In the future, I will grow my own vegetables.

In the future, I will medically transition, and my body will look nothing like it looks now. Some parts of my body will retain their softness; other parts will be stronger, harder, and every part of me, every inch, will glisten like raw obsidian.

//

For my own survival, I have to believe I have a future.

I wish I could have seen Alisha B. Wormsley's famous billboard *There Are Black People in the Future* when it was first installed in 2017, before it became a rallying cry or a shorthand for hope. To have experienced it as one single breath that inspires the next.

The original billboard lived in East Liberty, a neighborhood in Pittsburgh that I've never visited, and so I do not know its textures or its edges, the people who defined it and those who attempt to redefine it; but every American neighborhood is remarkable and unremarkable in that their histories overlap. So when I imagine what it would have been like to see the original art piece, the street is always empty, free of people and cars and the noises that are produced by them—and this is not a failure of my imagination, I don't think, or a vagueness that needs correction, rather a state of mind I'm trying to achieve, I think, a meditation.

In my imagination, I am alone, as I am often alone on walks. I am wearing a comfortable sweater and breathable pants and shoes that are beginning to fall apart. The weather is cool but not obnoxiously so. The sky is a deep black, throbbing, like my skin on the nights when I don't know how to soothe it. There is a streetlight—for how else am I to see where I'm headed—and its amber glow befriends a sadness in me that I rarely acknowledge.

I would probably be preoccupied—as I'm often ruminating on the things I should have said, the people I should have loved more responsibly—which is to say I would feel something adjacent to loneliness, the contentment of my solitude mixed with the sincere desire for me not to need so much of it.

At some point, I break away from my thoughts. Instead of looking behind me, I look up. And there it is in the sky: a beacon and a reminder that I'm never really alone. Bold, white letters on a big, black backdrop. A statement so simple I'm surprised that I needed those words to be said at all. And that surprise is what will break me—or rather the surprise breaks apart the pain I've been suffering and sets it ablaze so another feeling can be born anew. And suddenly, for the briefest respite, my future is a foregone conclusion, and not just an aspiration.

By the time I did see the billboard in person, or at least an iteration of it, it was at the Oakland Museum of California a year or two into the COVID pandemic. And it wasn't so much a billboard as it was very large words printed on a very wide wall near the museum's entrance. There were white round tables and white slatted chairs, most of which were empty except for a middle-aged white guy looking down at his phone. And it was sunny. And I was with my partner. And I was alive, which should have made me feel grateful when so many people were not, but at that point in time, the future just seemed so bleak, I couldn't even bear to look at those words—for what future would my people even be living?

Every day that year, I was trying to write my way back into life, back into the optimism that had helped me survive childhood, and every day I was never quite succeeding. I wouldn't say that the work rang hollow, just that I was hollow and afraid of what the future had in store for me (of whether I could even survive that future when my past, that childhood, had already been so utterly painful).

Now, after Trump's reelection, I can appreciate both experiences of this art—the imagined and the real—as imperatives for survival. This is the cycle of living. We hope. We dream. We struggle. We grieve. We hope. We dream. We struggle. We grieve. We hope. We dream.

//

During my quietest evenings, when I am alone and my skin feels so thin that even the wind bruises it, I wish only to be alive in the future.

Because what a privilege it'll be to grow old—to celebrate my seventieth birthday in my backyard with my friends who are family, my sister and her partner, my partner (or partners), my children (and perhaps their children if they choose to bring their own little ones into this world).

Around us the hills will be scorched from the most recent wildfire season, the fields bitter and black but not unloving.

(The earth, I have to believe, will find a way to survive despite the harm we have done to it—just as I have survived and survive and survive.)

My family and I will commune in the small garden that we have grown with our bare hands—the bulbs of lettuce, our black beans, the few raspberries we protected from the ravenous birds, pockets of lavender and sweet tomatoes and potatoes. The air will be cool and forgiving. I will feel strong and loved, not for the first or last time in my life (and won't that be the best blessing), and while my family laughs and exchanges stories that detail all the soft, messy parts of me, I will be distracted, thinking again about this beautiful, cruel world and how I've always wished to leave it in a better state than I received it, but how I've always known, quite acutely, that I will fail and I have already failed in most of what I aim to do.

That is for my children to achieve, I say out loud, interrupting everyone's revelry, and my adult children will groan and roll their eyes lovingly because I am always doing that these days, sharing only the last sentence of the epic paragraphs I've written inside my head.

In this way, I am realizing the future is both a noun and a verb. Some futures are only possible if I step toward them. To say out loud what I want out of this one precious life with which I have been blessed (and burdened), and then to reach for those things, really reach, with the full force of my stupid sentimental heart.

ACKNOWLEDGMENTS

When I approached Halimah Marcus with the idea to publish a limited series of essays written by trans and gender-nonconforming writers of color on *Electric Literature*, the first thing she said was "yes," and the second thing she said was "How can I help?" Her leadership, her professional partnership, and her friendship paved the way for me to make this series, and then this book, happen. For every success of *Both/And*, she remains by my side, uplifting and amplifying my work. My gratitude is immeasurable.

Thank you to my agent, Robert Guinsler, and Electric Lit's agent, Sarah Bowlin, who trumpeted their love for this project and created a whirlwind of support.

Working with Rakesh Satyal as my editor and with his assistant, Ryan Amato, has been a dream come true. They have been incredible advocates and advisors in stewarding this project through its publication process, always offering wisdom alongside encouraging words. We wouldn't be here without them, as well as the rest of the HarperOne team.

To Electric Lit's board of directors, who so keenly have our back through good times and bad: Andy Hunter, Sara Nelson,

Michael Cunningham, Nicole Cliffe, Meredith Talusan, and Deesha Philyaw, thank you for always being in our corner.

To our staff, all of whom have taken on extra work to support me as I've worked on this project—Wynter Miller, Katie Henken Robinson, Jo Lou, Kelly Luce, Willem Marx, and Preety Sidhu; and interns Courtney DuChene, Skylar Miklus, Jalen G. Jones, Vivienne Germain, Kyla Walker, Chris Vanjonack, Kristina Busch, Laura Schmitt, Nzinga Temu, Marina Leigh, Lisa Zhuang, and Eliza Browning—thank you for your patience.

Thank you to Adonis Brown, who worked with me exclusively on this project and helped me curate the original series. Thank you to Jennifer Baker, Michele Filgate, and R. O. Kwon for offering key insights and advice on the work of curating and publishing an anthology.

My enormous heartfelt gratitude to the writers who appeared in the online series, whose words laid the groundwork for the scope of this project: Logan Hoffman-Smith, Leo D. Martinez, M. Jesuthasan, Stacy Nathaniel Jackson, Fayth Tan, Ching-In Chen, Summer Tao, H. P. Cilgin, and 12:41, thank you for trusting me, and *EL*, with your precious work. It has been our honor to publish it.

And to the writers who make up this book: Addie Tsai, Vanessa Angélica Villarreal, Peppermint, Kai Cheng Thom, Jonah Wu, Gabrielle Bellot, Akwaeke Emezi, Meredith Talusan, Denny, Edgar Gomez, Tanaïs, Autumn Fourkiller, Raquel Willis, Caro De Robertis, Zeyn Joukhadar, Kaia Ball, and A. L. Major—I will continue shouting your names from the rooftops.

It takes a lot of bravery to be visible right now as a trans person; I am indebted to, and in awe of, your bravery, and that of those who came before us.

CONTRIBUTORS

Kaia Ball crafts fiction with a scientist's attention, nonfiction with an artist's panache, and poetry like a love story to life itself. Their art strives to honor the vitality of building, sharing, and existing in community. Find their work on soup, pigeons, and trans joy at kaia-ball.com and @kaiaballwrites.bsky.social.

Gabrielle Bellot is a staff writer for *Literary Hub*. Formerly, she served as the head instructor at Catapult's Classes department, as well as a contributing editor for the *Catapult* online magazine. Before the magazine department shuttered, she wrote a regular column for *Catapult* called "Wander, Woman," which examined books, the body, memory, and more. One of these columns, "The Curious Language of Grief," was a notable essay in *The Best American Essays 2021*. In 2023, she was a reader for the 10th annual Vulture Festival's "Feminist as F*ck" event in Los Angeles, arranged by Roxane Gay and Amber Tamblyn, alongside Amber, R. O. Kwon, Nafissa Thompson-Spires, and Kirsten Vangsness. She is the author of *My Year of Psychedelics: Lessons on Better Living* (2024), one of the inaugural works in Roxane Gay's "Roxane Gay &" series. Bellot is also a certified transformational coach with a focus on psychedelic integration, shadow work, and self-growth. She runs Bliss Witch, her own coaching practice. If you'd like to learn more about her coaching or schedule a session, you can visit her separate coaching site at https://gabriellebellot .com/writingcoach.

Denny is a writer, actor, and musician currently working as the LGBTQ communities reporter at Reckon News. She appeared in *Pose* and *New Amsterdam* and will be appearing in Apple TV's upcoming murder mystery series *City on Fire*, an adaptation of Garth Risk Hallberg's novel. Her writing has appeared in *Allure*, *Paper*, and other outlets. Her *New York Times* "Modern Love" essay "He Made Affection Feel Simple" was published in June 2021.

Caro De Robertis, a writer of Uruguayan origins, is the author of *So Many Stars: An Oral History of Trans, Nonbinary, Gender-queer, and Two-Spirit People of Color*, as well as *The Palace of Eros*, a finalist for the Octavia Butler CALIBA Golden Poppy Award; *The President and the Frog*, a finalist for the PEN/Faulkner Award and the PEN/Jean Stein Book Award; *Cantoras*, winner of a Stonewall Book Award and a Reading Women Award, a finalist for the Kirkus Prize and a Lambda Literary Award, and a *New York Times* Editors' Choice; *The Gods of Tango*, winner of a Stonewall Book Award; *Perla*; and the international bestseller *The Invisible Mountain*, which received Italy's Rhegium Julii Prize. Their books have been translated into seventeen languages and have received numerous other honors, including a fellowship from the National Endowment for the Arts and the John

Dos Passos Prize for Literature, which they were the first openly nonbinary person to receive. De Robertis is a professor at San Francisco State University and lives in Oakland, California, with their two children.

Akwaeke Emezi is the author of *Pet*, a finalist for the National Book Award for Young People's Literature, a Walter Honor Book, and a Stonewall Honor Book; the *New York Times* bestseller *The Death of Vivek Oji*, which was a finalist for the Dylan Thomas Prize, the Los Angeles Times Book Prize, and the PEN/Jean Stein Award; *Freshwater*, which was named a New York Times Notable Book and shortlisted for the PEN/Hemingway Award, the New York Public Library Young Lions Fiction Award, the Lambda Literary Award, and the Center for Fiction's First Novel Prize; and, most recently, *Dear Senthuran: A Black Spirit Memoir*. Their debut poetry collection, *Content Warning: Everything*, published in 2022. Selected as a 5 Under 35 honoree by the National Book Foundation, they are based in liminal spaces.

Autumn Fourkiller is a writer and mystic from the "early death capital of the world." She is currently at work on a novel about Indigenous identity, the Olympics, and climate change. A 2022 Ann Friedman Weekly Fellow, her work can be found in *Atlas Obscura*, *Majuscule*, *Longreads*, and elsewhere. You can follow her newsletter, *Dream Interpretation for Dummies*, on Substack.

Edgar Gomez is a queer NicaRican writer born and raised in Florida. He is the author of the memoir *High-Risk Homosexual*, winner of the American Book Award, a Stonewall Book Award–

Israel Fishman Non-Fiction Award, and the Lambda Literary Award. Their sophomore book, *Alligator Tears,* was released in February 2025. A graduate of the University of California's MFA program, Gomez has written for the *Los Angeles Times, Poets & Writers, Lit Hub, New York Magazine,* and more. He has received fellowships from the New York Foundation for the Arts, the National Endowment for the Arts, and Black Mountain Institute. He lives between New York and Puerto Rico. Find him across social media: @OtroEdgarGomez.

Zeyn Joukhadar is the author of the novels *The Thirty Names of Night,* which won the Lambda Literary Award and the Stonewall Book Award, and *The Map of Salt and Stars,* which won the Middle East Book Award and was a Goodreads Choice Awards and Wilbur Smith Adventure Writing Prize finalist. His work has appeared or is forthcoming in *Salon, The Paris Review, [PANK],* and elsewhere and has been included in anthologies such as *Kink, This Arab Is Queer, Letters to a Writer of Color,* and others. He has been twice nominated for the Pushcart Prize. Joukhadar guest-edited *Mizna*'s 2020 "Queer + Trans Voices" issue, serves on the board of the Radius of Arab American Writers (RAWI), and mentors emerging writers of color with the Periplus Collective.

A. L. Major, originally from the Bahamas, has received fellowships and residencies from Aspen Words, Tin House, Baldwin for the Arts, and Monson Arts. Their work has appeared in *Vice* magazine and *Subtropics.* They earned their MFA in fiction from the University of Michigan, where they were also awarded a Hopwood Novel Award. They are currently working on their debut novel, *Every Day You Wake You Raise the Dead*. AL is the director of online programs at Tin House.

Miss Peppermint is an American actress, singer, songwriter, television personality, drag queen, and activist. She is best known from the nightlife scene and, in 2017, as the runner-up on the ninth season of *RuPaul's Drag Race*.

Meredith Talusan received a Creative Capital Award and MacDowell Fellowship for fiction in 2023; her stories appear or are forthcoming in *Guernica*, *Kenyon Review*, *Boston Review*, *Epoch*, *The Rumpus*, *Grand*, *Catapult*, and *BLR*. Her debut memoir, *Fairest*, was a 2020 Lambda Literary Award finalist and named a best book of the year by multiple venues. She has contributed to ten other books and written articles for *The New York Times*, *The Atlantic*, *The Guardian*, and *Wired*, among many other outlets. She has received journalism awards from GLAAD, the Society of Professional Journalists, and NLGJA: The Association of LGBTQ+ Journalists. She is also the founding executive editor and current contributing editor at *them*, Condé Nast's LGBTQ+ digital platform.

Tanaïs is a writer, an artist, and the perfumer behind the independent beauty and fragrance house TANAÏS. They are the author of *In Sensorium: Notes for My People*, winner of the 2022 Kirkus Prize for Nonfiction, and *Bright Lines*, a novel.

Kai Cheng Thom is a writer, performance artist, and community healer in Toronto. She is the author of the novel *Fierce Femmes* *and Notorious Liars: A Dangerous Trans Girl's Confabulous Memoir*, the essay collection *I Hope We Choose Love: A Trans Girl's Notes at the End of the World* (an American Library Association Stonewall Honor Book), the poetry collection *a place called No Homeland* (an American Library Association Stonewall Honor Book), and the children's picture books *From the Stars in the Sky to the Fish in the Sea*, illustrated by Kai Yun Ching and Wai-Yant Li, and *For Laika, the Dog Who Learned the Names of the Stars*, illustrated by Kai Yun Ching. Kai Cheng won the Writers' Trust of Canada's Dayne Ogilvie Prize for LGBTQ Emerging Writers in 2017.

Addie Tsai is a biracial Asian artist and writer who teaches at William & Mary. Addie collaborated with Dominic Walsh Dance Theater on *Victor Frankenstein* and *Camille Claudel*, among others. They are the author of *Dear Twin* and *Unwieldy Creatures*, which was a Shirley Jackson Award finalist for Best Novel. She is the features and reviews editor, as well as fiction coeditor, for *Anomaly*, and the founding editor in chief for *just femme & dandy*.

Vanessa Angélica Villarreal is the author of *Magical/Realism: Essays on Music, Memory, Fantasy, and Borders* (2024), longlisted for the National Book Award, and *Beast Meridian* (2017), recipient of a 2019 Whiting Award and a Kate Tufts Discovery Award nomination, and winner of the John A. Robertson Award for Best First Book of Poetry from the Texas Institute of Letters. She is a 2021 National Endowment for the Arts Fellow and holds a doctorate in English literature and creative writing from the University of Southern California in Los Angeles, where she lives with her son.

Raquel Willis is an African American writer, editor, and transgender rights activist. She is a former national organizer for the Transgender Law Center and the former executive editor of *Out Magazine*, and she currently serves as the director of communications for the Ms. Foundation for Women. Her debut memoir, *The Risk It Takes to Bloom*, was released in 2023.

Jonah Wu is a nonbinary and transmasculine Chinese American fiction writer and essayist. Their work can be found in *Longleaf Review*, *beestung*, *Jellyfish Review*, *Bright Wall/Dark Room*, *The Seventh Wave*, *smoke and mold*, and the *Los Suelos* anthology. They are a three-time Pushcart nominee and winner of Brave New Weird: The Best New Weird Horror of 2022. You can follow them on X or Instagram @rabblerouses.

ABOUT THE EDITOR AND ELECTRIC LITERATURE

About the Editor

Denne Michele Norris is the editor in chief of Electric Literature, where she became the first Black, openly transgender woman to helm a major literary publication. A 2021 Out100 Honoree, her writing has been supported by MacDowell, Tin House, and the Kimbilio for Black Fiction, and has appeared in *McSweeney's*, *American Short Fiction*, and *Zora*. She is the former fiction editor of both *Apogee Journal* and *The Rumpus*, a cohost of the critically acclaimed podcast *Food 4 Thot*, and a mentor to emerging writers of color with the Periplus Collective. Her debut novel, *When the Harvest Comes*, was published in April 2025. She lives in New York City.

About Electric Literature

Electric Literature is a nonprofit digital publisher with the mission to make literature more exciting, relevant, and inclusive.